DISCOVER THE HO...
CAN SLIM YO...

Leading medical doctor Sandra Cab... weight where you do—*and what you can do about it.* Her revolutionary diet for weight loss gives you the tools to drop pounds easily and stay the shape you love—forever! Discover:

- Your specific body type—lymphatic, android, gynecoid, or thyroid.
- Which foods you crave, which to avoid, and why your body stores the fat, flab, and cellulite where it does.
- An easy, never-feel-hungry diet individualized for your hormones that's heart-healthy, packed with vitamins, and includes soothing herbal teas.
- Dozens of low-fat, low-calorie recipes, specific eating plans for each body type, and toning and shaping exercises.
- The secrets of turning on your metabolism to start melting pounds away—today!

NO DANGEROUS FAD FOOD!
NO EXTREME REGIMENS!
AN ALL-NATURAL APPROACH
THAT IS GENTLE
ON YOUR SYSTEM AND
IMMUNE BOOSTING, TOO!

THE BODY-SHAPING DIET

Dr. Sandra Cabot

WARNER BOOKS

A Time Warner Company

This program is not intended as a substitute for medical advice. As
with any diet book, you are advised to consult regularly with
your health care professional in matters which may require diagnosis
or medical attention. This book contains numerous case histories.
In order to preserve the privacy of the people involved, their names
have been changed.

All information contained in this book regarding brand-name
products is based on research by the authors, which is accurate
as of April 1, 1994.

First published in 1993 by Women's Health Advisory Service,
Australia.
Copyright © 1993 by Dr. Sandra Cabot
All rights reserved.

Visit our Web site at
http://pathfinder.com/twep

Warner Books, Inc., 1271 Avenue of the Americas,
New York, NY 10020
A Time Warner Company

Printed in the United States of America
Originally published in hardcover by Warner Books, Inc.
First Printed in Paperback: April, 1996
10 9 8 7 6 5 4 3 2

Cartoons by Karen Barbouttis
Body shape illustrations by Vilma Topolovic
Exercise illustrations by Vilma Topolovic
Book design by Giorgetta Bell McRee
Cover design by Don Munson
Cover photography by James Pozarik

DEDICATION

This book is dedicated to the late Vicki Petersen, undoubtedly the most brilliant and witty Australian health writer I have ever known. For those who were fortunate enough to know Vicki life will never be the same. I first met her in Sydney in 1981, when I was starting to put pen to paper. She was at this time a prolific journalist for many top women's magazines including *Vogue*, *Harper's Bazaar*, *Nature and Health* and *Woman's Day* and wrote with such panache and enthusiasm that one could always recognize the typical stamp of a Petersen article.

She had written several internationally best-selling books, including *Whole Food Catalogue*, *Eat Your Way to Health*, *Strategies of the Champions*, *Food Combining* and a travel book on Australia, and had so many plans to write future books on health and well-being. The next two off the press were to be cookbooks called *The Lean Green Mamma's Cookbook* and *Be Happy Not Hungry*.

Whoever would have thought that this brilliant and powerful woman was to become a victim of anorexia nervosa.

It came as a huge shock to all who knew and read her when she died in one of Sydney's public hospitals on August 29, 1992, with kidney and liver failure as a result of malnutrition.

It is a tragedy that it takes the untimely death of such a tremendous woman as Vicki Petersen to bring home the message that we need to do more to help women with eating disorders. We need to do more for women caught in the lonely battle against eating disorders and obesity and the associated chronic health problems and dangers that they incur. We can change our body weight and shape in a scientific, safe and enjoyable way without becoming neurotically unhappy and caught in the superficial and stereotyped expectations that today's society projects. Obesity and eating disorders are a state of mind reflecting a loss of balance in our mental, emotional and physical lives. They are not primarily a physical disease like a cold or arthritis, which can be alleviated by treating the symptoms. We need to dig deeper and find the hidden mental agenda of negativity, poor self-image and loss of confidence.

The book *The Body-Shaping Diet* has been written to overcome these negative aspects in our mind that keep us trapped in obesity or an eating disorder. It is not just another hip and thigh diet, but rather a way of eating for a vital mind and body. *The Body-Shaping Diet* will rebalance your hormonal and metabolic system specifically for your body shape. It will stimulate your entire physical and mental physiology, increasing your energy levels and vitality, thus overcoming all the negative obstacles in your mind that have previously held you back and told you that you cannot be slim and healthy and feel good about yourself. You no longer have to feel that you are alone in your struggle to maintain a healthy body weight if you use this book as a vehicle to travel with you and guide and support you in your journey to total health.

C O N T E N T S

B O D Y   T Y P E S

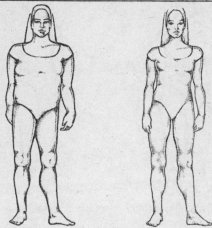

Android body shape (left) overweight, (right) ideal weight

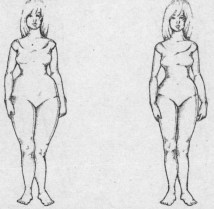

Gynecoid body shape (left) overweight, (right) ideal weight

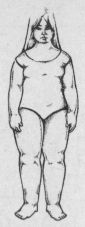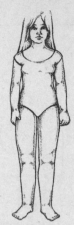

Lymphatic body shape (left) overweight, (right) ideal weight

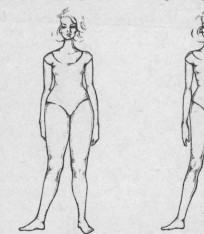

Thyroid body shape (left) overweight, (right) ideal weight

INTRODUCTION

The last fifteen years of my life have been spent working with women suffering with chronic health problems, hormonal imbalance and excess weight. I have researched these areas extensively and have a vast experience in investigating and treating women in a clinical context. Thanks to technology and sophisticated tools of diagnosis, it is now easy to scientifically pinpoint the type of hormonal imbalance present. We can now tell from blood hormone assays whether your numerous glands, such as the pituitary, thyroid, adrenals and ovaries, are under- or overactive. It is possible to treat these imbalances with hormone replacement therapy using natural types of hormones and for this we can lay our gratitude firmly at the door of modern medicine.

However, when it comes to a large array of chronic health complaints, weight excess being included here, the tools of modern medicine and chemical pharmacology often provide only partial or temporary solutions. Thankfully, for the last twenty years I have researched nutritional medicine, an interest of mine that started way back in medical school. The science and art of treating diseases and obesity with special diets, vitamins, minerals, amino acids and essential fatty acids is a tremendously satisfying healing tool for any doctor.

It is a form of healing that I am able to utilize and write about with authority because of my background and my years of clinical experience with thousands of patients who were not responding to conventional medicine alone. If you are battling with a weight problem and its associated health complaints, I assure you that you can overcome them with a change of diet and specific nutritional strategies—all it takes is the decision to start. Make it today! The first three months is the hardest phase but after six months you will be feeling and looking much better and after twelve months on the Body-Shaping Diet you will feel and look the best you can possibly be!

The Body-Shaping Diet has been followed by many of my patients for many different reasons. Some have used it to lower their blood pressure, eradicate candida and allergies, reduce headaches or just improve their general health. Others have used it just to lose weight while some have stuck to it for years in a committed effort to change their body shape. No one has a perfect body and we all have room for improvement. Some women become really hung up or unhappy about a part of themselves, so much so that they allow it to erode their self-esteem and personality. I try to show women that they must first accept themselves as a unique individual with a unique beauty. The next step is to make the best of what you've got right now, today! Don't let life pass you by! You should never change yourself just to please another but rather do it for yourself first. The Body-Shaping Diet and exercise programs will make it possible for you to achieve your desired weight or to change your shape if you so wish, so that you can feel really great about being you. Whether you want to look sexier, fitter, slimmer, more sporty, more or less shapely or simply glow with health, the Body-Shaping Diet can do it for you.

Diagram 1

ENDOCRINE GLANDS AND THEIR HORMONES

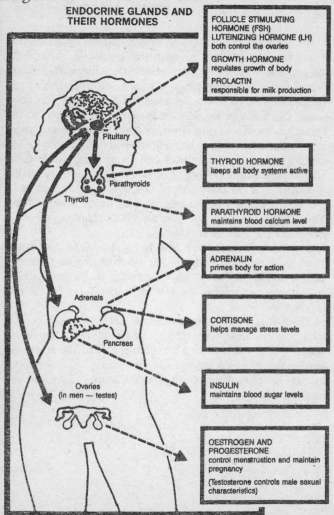

FOLLICLE STIMULATING HORMONE (FSH)
LUTEINIZING HORMONE (LH)
both control the ovaries

GROWTH HORMONE
regulates growth of body

PROLACTIN
responsible for milk production

THYROID HORMONE
keeps all body systems active

PARATHYROID HORMONE
maintains blood calcium level

ADRENALIN
primes body for action

CORTISONE
helps manage stress levels

INSULIN
maintains blood sugar levels

OESTROGEN AND PROGESTERONE
control menstruation and maintain pregnancy

(Testosterone controls male sexual characteristics)

Pituitary

Parathyroids

Thyroid

Adrenals

Pancreas

Ovaries
(in men — testes)

WHAT IS THE
BODY-SHAPING DIET?

It is a unique and scientifically designed eating plan for life. There are four different eating plans specifically tailored for the four different body shapes of women. All women fall into one of these four categories—gynecoid, android, thyroid and lymphatic—which you will understand as you read this book (page 15). Each of the four body shapes, if exposed to the wrong types of foods on a consistent basis, may become obese in different areas of their body. Some body shapes can eat so-called fattening foods without becoming obese while other body shapes cannot. Similarly, no one simple calorie-restricted diet works for all body shapes and it is more important to change the sources of the calories than to just restrict them. These differences apply because each body shape has a unique metabolic and hormonal makeup.

The Body-Shaping Diet matches your unique shape and hormonal makeup to the foods that will stimulate and rebalance your metabolism. This is what makes the Body-Shaping Diet so effective, not only in the first few months, but for the rest of your life.

There will be no need to follow restrictive diets or feel hungry, weak and deprived, because by following the Body-Shaping Diet you will feel satisfied, energetic and positively rebalanced. What's more you will lose weight where you want to, thus sculpting your physique into a more streamlined and balanced form.

ARE YOU READY TO MAKE A COMMITMENT TO THE BODY-SHAPING DIET?

- Are you ready to lose weight efficiently?
- Are you ready to reshape your body into a form that pleases you?
- Are you ready to tone and firm up and lose all your cellulite?
- Are you ready to feel feminine and more sexually alive?
- Are you ready to reduce your hormonal imbalances?
- Are you ready to feel more energetic, productive and increase your zest for life?
- Are you ready to improve your general health and well-being and boost your immune system?

If your answers are Yes—you are ready to make the Body-Shaping Diet commitment!

Congratulations on your decision to look and feel the best you possibly can. The Body-Shaping Diet will streamline your body shape and give you the key to weight control, better health and vitality.

WHY HASN'T SOMEBODY TOLD YOU THIS BEFORE?

The subject of women's hormones, or gynecological endocrinology as it is called in medical terminology, is a new specialty in medicine and doctors are only beginning to understand its powerful influence in our daily lives. The realization that our body shape and weight are linked to our dominant hormonal gland is also a new breakthrough, with exciting and practical implications for women with excess weight.

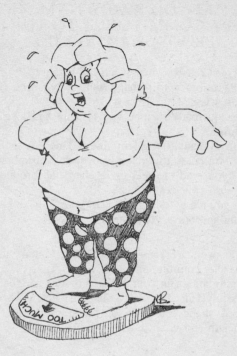

   For the first time ever we can now change our body shape and weight by rebalancing and fine-tuning the hormonal system through diet, nutritional supplements, exercise and, if necessary, hormone therapy.

   The old-fashioned simplistic way of losing weight through restrictive dieting and heavy exercise may work for some, but not for all. Furthermore, in the long term 95 percent of women who lose weight through restrictive low-calorie dieting will regain their undesirable weight. They will subject themselves to dangers such as extreme weight cycling, anemia, loss of muscle tissue, increased risk of osteoporosis and mineral imbalances. In contrast, the Body-Shaping Diet avoids unnecessary pain and hardship, does not put you at any risk and is guaranteed to work in the long term.

For all body shapes we have a tailor-made program of exercises to redistribute fat and muscle tissue and help remove stubborn fat deposits and cellulite. These exercises complement the Body-Shaping Diet (see page 281).

Investing our resources into our bodies is like investing our money. When and how we do it is crucial and in both endeavors it is vital to get the best professional advice. The Body-Shaping Diet ensures that your valuable resources of time and effort will be rewarded by basing our program on many years of clinical experience and research.

HOW THE BODY-SHAPING DIET WORKS ON THE CELLULAR LEVEL

To achieve weight loss and/or fat redistribution, we need to stimulate the metabolism or chemical processes within our fat cells. The metabolic rate of our body is the rate at which the body cells convert food energy into physical (kinetic) energy. The metabolic rate of an individual appears to be the most important determinant of body weight. Those with a slow or sluggish metabolic rate gain weight most rapidly and lose weight most slowly. The Body-Shaping Diet is designed to stimulate the metabolic rate of each fat cell by providing it with the correct proportions of nutrients, vitamins, minerals, water and hormones. This enables you not only to burn food calories at a faster rate, but facilitates the breakdown and/or redistribution of stubborn inactive fat deposits. Thus, weight loss and body reshaping becomes quicker, easier and, if you stick to the Body-Shaping Diet, long lasting.

Let's don the cap of a scientist for a moment and take a look at a fat cell under the microscope—see diagram 2. As

Diagram 2

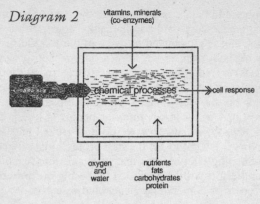

A FAT CELL

you can see the raw materials required for the chemical processes within each fat cell are hormones, vitamins, minerals,
oxygen, fats, carbohydrates and protein. If these raw materials
are out of balance—say, for example, too many sex hormones,
not enough vitamins and minerals, not enough oxygen and too
much saturated fat—then the inner chemical processes of the
fat cells do not occur efficiently and we have a reduction in
the metabolic rate. If this continues, weight gain is sure to
result, with accumulations of sluggish, underactive fat cells
appearing. Here we have the microscopic genesis of cellulite
and layers and ridges of unsightly fat.

You can now understand why it is vital to follow an eating
plan that works on each individual fat cell if you are really
going to change your body weight and shape in an efficient
and lasting way. The Body-Shaping Diet will do this by
providing each fat cell with the correct proportions of vitamins, minerals, fats, protein, carbohydrates and water.

In addition, the Body-Shaping Diet will rebalance the
cellular metabolism specifically for each of the four different
body shapes—android, gynecoid, thyroid and lymphatic.
The metabolism of the fat cells is different in each of the

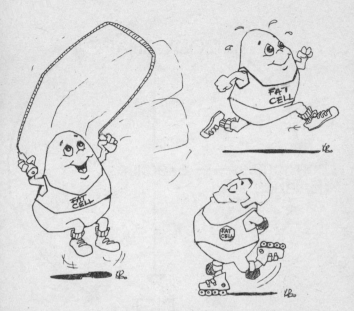

four body shapes and each shape requires a unique balance of vitamins, minerals, fats, protein and carbohydrates. When the correct balance of these nutrients for each body shape is supplied in the diet, we not only stimulate the metabolism of each fat cell but also achieve a rebalancing of the hormonal (endocrine) system. It is this latter effect that promotes the redistribution of body fat so that the body shape can begin to change in a way that pleases us—that is, more streamlined and balanced from head to toe.

It is the missing links between **body shape—diet—hormonal balance** that are so vital and have previously prevented women from changing their body shape. Of course, exercise is important too, and you can see from diagram 3 how all these factors influence each other. Standard calorie-

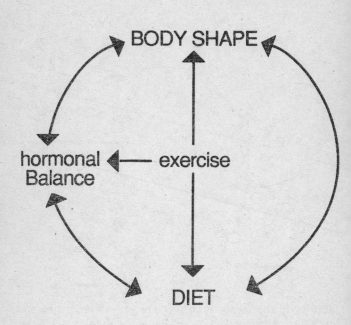

Diagram 3

restricted diets are limited—they only enable you to lose weight temporarily, but don't produce an overall balancing and redistribution of body fat. The Body-Shaping Diet and exercise program is a safe and effective permanent way to change your body shape and weight because it fills in the missing links.

PART ONE

WHAT SHAPE ARE YOU?

How to Recognize Your Body Shape

To fit yourself into one of the four female body shapes look at the diagrams beginning on page 18 and compare yourself to these, full frontal and sideways, while standing naked in front of the mirror. Choose the body shape that most closely resembles your own.

The most common types of body shapes are android and gynecoid, in approximately equal numbers (although race does influence the relative proportions of each body shape in a given population). The lymphatic and thyroid types are less common body shapes.

Your body shape is genetically determined (inherited); the basic musculoskeletal structure and the relative proportions of various body parts are different for each body shape. Your height and/or weight do not determine your body shape or type. For example, you can be a thin short or fat short or thin tall or fat tall android body shape. The underlying body proportions and musculoskeletal structure of a given shape will be similar in every individual with that shape, although their outward appearance can vary greatly. In particular, all androids have the characteristics of a small narrow pelvis and hips, muscular limbs, and a trunk (torso) that is broad and straight up and down in shape. (By the way, the vast majority of men are android in shape.) All the other body shapes—namely gynecoid, lymphatic and thyroid—can also be tall or short, fat or thin, while retaining the underlying body proportions and musculoskeletal structures that determine the respective body shapes.

THE ANDROID SHAPE

This shape is characterized by a strong, thickset skeletal frame with large shoulders, a large rib cage and muscular limbs. The neck, chest and abdomen are rather thick and the pelvis is small so that android women are relatively straight up and down. They lack feminine curves and have muscular buttocks and powerful muscular thighs. The pelvis and buttocks do not curve outward very much below a rather thick waist.

Android women are somewhat masculine in shape and often make good athletes in sports requiring strength and staying power, such as bodybuilding, swimming and long-distance running. They may be told that they resemble their fathers or brothers and yet these women are very attractive and glow with health. The bones in their limbs, hands and feet are large and they have more muscle mass and less fat tissue than most women unless they become overweight.

If weight gain occurs, fat is deposited in the upper part of the body—above the pelvis. This produces a thickening of the neck, trunk, waist and abdomen and gives rise to the term "apple-shaped obesity." The first part of the body to gain weight in android types is the abdomen and as fat accumulates around the front part of the waistline, this protuberant abdomen

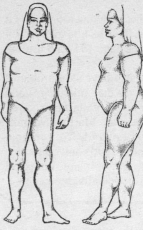

ANDROID
BODY SHAPE
OVERWEIGHT

ANDROID
BODY SHAPE
IDEAL WEIGHT

may produce the impression of a potbelly or pregnancy. Despite this, the hips remain narrow and the legs retain their shapely muscular form. If weight gain continues, fat will be deposited above the hips and around the trunk (torso), producing the appearance of handlebars above the hips and spare tires around the trunk. These are not flattering terms but nevertheless illustrate easily the general thickening of the upper body that occurs in android types as they gain excessive weight. The breasts may be small, medium or large in size and with excessive weight gain may become huge due to their large fat content. This is part of the apple-shaped obesity typical of android types.

Android-shaped persons tend to put on weight easily, especially at middle age, if they are inactive and eat a normal Western diet that contains too much fat and salt for their body types. This can be avoided by following the android diet (see page 104) and leading an active lifestyle.

The android woman may also have skin problems such as excess facial and body hair (hirsutism) and acne as a result of her higher levels of male hormones.

Examples of android women are Martina Navratilova, Madonna and Cindy Crawford. Yes, android types are much in vogue in the 1990s and epitomize the powerful beauty and strength of many successful and healthy women. For further details, see page 44.

THE GYNECOID SHAPE

This shape is characterized by a pear shape, with the body flaring outward toward the hips and thighs. The buttocks are curved and rounded and the thighs are curved outward laterally and may touch together on the inside or medial aspect. The bottom has a tendency to droop downward (posterially) over the back of the thighs. The waist is tapered and smaller than the hips, giving a feminine appearance. The breasts are variably sized and may be small to large. The shoulders are small to moderate in size. Typical measurements for a gynecoid woman are 39″, 29″, 43″.

The bones of the arms and legs are feminine with tapered, fine forearms, wrists, shins and ankles. Even if obesity occurs, the forearms and shins remain relatively fine and slim, with fat tissue accumulating firstly on the thighs, buttocks, breasts and later over the lower abdomen in front of the pubic bones. The bones of the pelvic cavity are wide, thus giving rise

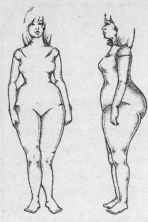

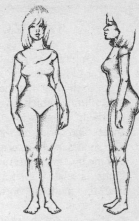

*GYNECOID
BODY SHAPE
OVERWEIGHT*

*GYNECOID
BODY SHAPE
IDEAL WEIGHT*

to the term "good childbearing hips." Many women fit into the gynecoid shape, which is logical as women have been designed to give birth to babies, with the rather large head coming first.

Gynecoid women are generally medium to short in height and occasionally can be quite tall, but in proportion to their trunk, their legs and arms are not as long as in thyroid shapes. Gynecoid women put on weight easily, especially around the bottom and upper thighs, if they don't take care with food combining (see page 55 for more details). Examples of famous gynecoid types include Marilyn Monroe and Elizabeth Taylor.

THE LYMPHATIC SHAPE

The lymphatic-shaped woman is characterized by a generalized thickening and puffiness of the body. This is due to the fact that she retains water easily, especially in her limbs, which gives her thick arms and legs with a straight up-and-down look along their length. The ankles and wrists are thick and puffy in appearance. The shoulders, breasts and rib cage are average in size and the abdomen protrudes in front. The trunk, like the limbs, is relatively straight up and down, with a thick waist and moderate outward curves on the buttocks and pelvic area.

The bones of the skeleton and the muscles are average in size and their shape is not clearly defined as they are covered by a thickish layer of fat and fluid. In other words it is difficult to see their bone structure and they are definitely not the bony type, which we find among thyroid-shaped women.

The thick straight up-and-down look comes from the accumulation of fluid and fat in the tissues under the skin (subcutaneous layer), which is evenly distributed over the bone and muscle structures. If a lymphatic woman becomes obese her fat will be distributed all over her body, in the legs, feet, arms, hands, buttocks, abdomen, trunk, neck and face. Lymphatic women have often been chubby since childhood and resemble a cupid or cuddly baby doll; most find that they gain weight easily.

Indeed, of all the body shapes, the lymphatic woman will gain weight the most easily as her metabolism is very slow. She will always be struggling with her weight if she consumes a normal Western diet. Two famous lymphatic-type women are Roseanne and Ella Fitzgerald. For further details, see page 65.

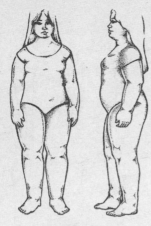

*LYMPHATIC
BODY SHAPE
OVERWEIGHT*

*LYMPHATIC
BODY SHAPE
IDEAL WEIGHT*

THE THYROID SHAPE

The thyroid woman is characterized by a narrow streamlined shape with long limbs and fine bones. The limbs are relatively long compared to the trunk. The long arms and legs produce a thoroughbred race-horse look. The breasts tend to be smallish although they may be moderate in size. Thyroid-shaped women are often tall, but even if they are not, they give the impression of being tall because of their long fine limbs. They have a somewhat boyish figure, with a narrow waist and generally only small curves on the buttocks and thighs. They move gracefully and may be athletes, especially sprinters or basketball players,

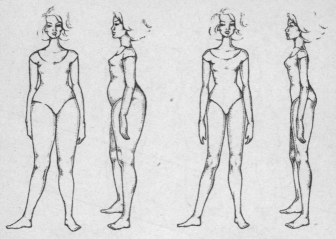

*THYROID
BODY SHAPE
OVERWEIGHT*

*THYROID
BODY SHAPE
IDEAL WEIGHT*

dancers or one of today's models. Twiggy and Jerry
Hall are examples of the thyroid shape.

Their fingers and toes are long and fine to match
their limbs and their necks are long and tend to be
narrow. They could be described as willowy, meaning
willow tree–like, and may have a fragile look about
them. Their bones are small to average in size and
the bone structure is clearly defined beneath a thin
layer of subcutaneous fat. They are often bony in
appearance, with their ribs and bony protuberances
(knobs) around their joints being very evident.

If weight gain occurs, fat is first deposited around
the abdomen and upper thighs with the upper part of
the body remaining slim. We call this body shape
thyroid because women with this body shape have a
high metabolic rate and do not put on weight easily.

It is associated with the thyroid gland because this gland controls the metabolic rate and is the dominant gland in thyroid people. Being a thyroid shape does not mean you have a problem with your thyroid gland, and, conversely, just because you may have a disease of your thyroid gland does not make you a thyroid-shaped person. Your body shape is always determined by your body proportions. For further details, see page 78.

CHAPTER TWO

WHY DO WE BECOME OVERWEIGHT?

It used to be thought that a person could not become overweight unless they consumed more energy in the form of calories than the amount of energy required to maintain and exercise the body. We now know that this is far too simplistic because obesity can occur from the interaction of increasing age, emotional imbalance, incorrect hormone therapy, underactive metabolic rate and incorrect food combining as well as the consumption of a diet that is wrong for your body shape. This will all be explained shortly.

It is interesting to note from diagram 4 that small people need fewer calories to maintain their weight than larger people. For example, a woman aged twenty-five years weighing 88 pounds needs only 1550 calories daily to maintain her body weight whereas a woman weighing 165 pounds at the same age requires 2400 calories daily. An intake of 500 calories a day less than the amount required to maintain body weight should lead to a weight loss of around 1 pound every week. Thus, you can see that a forty-five-year-old woman weighing 143 pounds could lose one pound each week on a 1600-**calorie** daily diet.

However, this **simple** balancing equation does not work for every woman! I have seen countless women who have

Diagram 4

CALORIES REQUIRED FOR MAINTENANCE OF VARIOUS BODY WEIGHTS

Weight	Calorie intake		
lbs	25 years	45 years	65 years
88	1550	1450	1400
99	1700	1600	1550
110	1800	1700	1650
121	1950	1850	1800
132	2050	1950	1900
143	2200	2100	2000
154	2300	2200	2100
165	2400	2300	2200

rigorously matched the calories they consumed to the number of calories they used up for body maintenance and exercise, only to find that they slowly continue to gain weight. They usually came to see me in a very confused and frustrated state and were often suffering from depression. Later I was able to reveal to them the reasons why they could not lose weight by explaining the factors affecting the metabolic rate of their fat cells (diagram 2 on page 10).

Let us review these reasons and how they thwart our well-meaning attempts to lose weight by calorie restriction alone.

1. INCREASING AGE. As we advance in years, the chemical processes or metabolic rate of our cells slows down. Thus, we gradually begin to burn calories at a slower rate. Many premenopausal and menopausal women will relate to this as they begin to develop a middle-aged spread around the abdomen.

This annoying tendency can be avoided by regular exer-

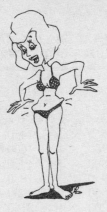

cise (at least forty minutes daily) and by reducing the amount of saturated fats in the diet. Foods that are high in saturated fats and must be avoided are: full-fat dairy products, fatty and processed meats, processed and take-out foods and fried foods. Older women should replace these undesirable foods with grains, cereals, legumes, lean meats, skim milk products, fresh fruit and vegetables.

Furthermore, as we age our cells become more dehydrated; in other words, they have a reduced water content. This causes a slower elimination of toxins and waste products from our cells, which results in sluggish chemical processes within the cells. To offset this poor metabolism, older women should increase their intake of water to 1 to 2 quarts daily and reduce their intake of coffee, sugary drinks, alcohol and salt.

By following these simple steps you will avoid becoming fat, matronly or middle-aged in appearance. Start well before the menopause so that it does not catch you unawares.

2. EMOTIONAL HUNGER. Many women are so-called comfort eaters. In other words, they may not really be hungry

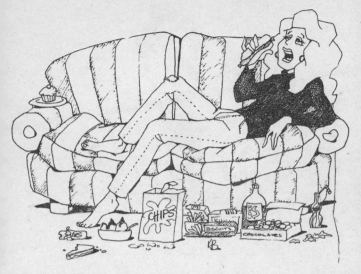

for food but they eat or drink when they feel depressed, helpless, powerless, rejected, lonely, ugly, poor, angry, frustrated or bored. In such cases, they are feeding their minds and souls with calories that only act as a temporary distraction or painkiller. Some women are afraid of their sexuality or of the opposite sex and subconsciously feel that by appearing overweight and undesirable they will not have to deal with these aspects of womanhood. As this method of self-defense is operating in the deeper subconscious mind, they may not be aware of the true nature of these fears, but only know that they somehow feel better when surrounded by a "suit of armor" in the form of a thick layer of fat. Such women may have been hurt or rejected in love affairs, sexually abused or be victims of incest.

Thus, obesity can be a symptom of emotional lack or imbalance and this should be looked for, especially if obesity is associated with anxiety, depression or mood disorders.

These problems can be overcome by working on your

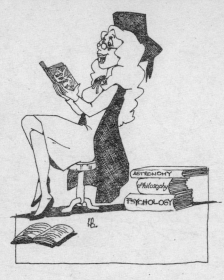

self-esteem and self-image. Very few of us are perfect and we can go a long way by accepting ourselves and making the best of our positive attributes. I see many women who do not appreciate the value of their own worth and need to increase self-esteem, self-confidence and assertiveness before dieting can become easy and effective.

Strategies that can fill the void of emotional hunger are many and varied and are not the subject of this book. However, there are a few worth mentioning:

a) Undertake counseling or psychotherapy to understand the reasons for your behavior. Read books on psychology, psychiatry and self-discovery. You can buy these or borrow them from a library.

b) Learn and practice meditation as it takes you back to the source of your being and enables you to know and love your inner self.

c) Be daring and do something you have always wanted to do but put on hold for a trillion reasons. Starting

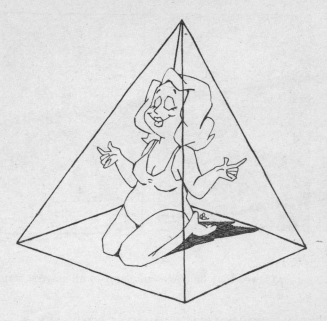

early and doing it little by little is better than delaying it for too long. Live your life as an exclamation, not as an explanation!

d) Don't become a doormat and slave to your partner, husband and children—tell them you need time to develop your own mind, body and soul. Take time for exercise, buying health foods and developing your intellect and creative talents. Many wives and mothers reach menopause and find themselves in the empty nest syndrome. They have forgotten themselves and wonder who they really are and what they are capable of. You will never know unless you try, so take my tip: Don't leave it until it's too late. Start developing your individuality, talents and desires way before menopause; other-

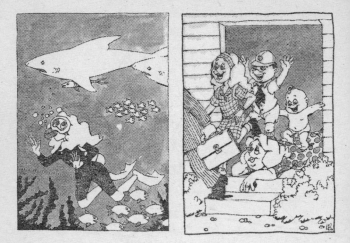

wise you may find yourself eating to fill up your empty nest.

3. INAPPROPRIATE HORMONE THERAPY.

In my experience approximately one in two women who start hormone replacement therapy (HRT) at menopause will gain a significant amount of weight. This is usually just about 4 to 5 pounds but it can occasionally be much more. This tendency can be avoided by asking your doctor to give you the natural brands of estrogen and progesterone instead of the synthetic brands of these hormones. Full details of natural estrogens and progesterone are found in my book *Smart Medicine for Menopause-Hormone Replacement Therapy and Its Natural Alternatives*. Quite a few menopausal women find that they need to reduce their dosage of hormone replacement therapy or, failing that, take their hormone replacement therapy in the form of the estrogen patch instead of tablets to avoid gaining weight.

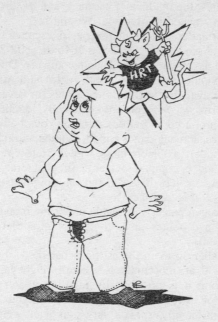

Generally speaking, heavier women require a smaller dose of hormone replacement therapy than lightweight or thin women. To avoid gaining weight they may need to take a smaller amount of progesterone, either by breaking the tablet in half or quarters or by taking it for a shorter time in each calendar month. Natural progesterone tablets or the seminatural progesterone called Duphaston (dydrogesterone) are less likely to put on weight than the synthetic progesterones. Synthetic progesterones are called progestagens and examples are norgestred, norethindrone and medroxyprogesterone acetate. In susceptible women such progestagens usually encourage weight gain. Natural progesterone tablets, suppositories and injections are available from the Women's International Pharmacy and Madison Pharmacy, both situated in Madison, Wisconsin.

For information on natural progesterone, contact Madison Pharmacy Associates, 1-800-558-7046 or 608-833-7046. Duphaston is made by the Dutch company Duphar and although popular in Europe, South Africa and Australia, it will not be available in the United States for several years. Natural forms of estrogen are chemically identical to the estrogens produced in various parts of your body such as your ovaries, adrenal glands and fat. Some natural brands of estrogen that are available in the United States are estradiol (Estrace) and estropipate (Ogen). Such natural forms of estrogen are far less likely to put on weight than are the stronger synthetic estrogens.

The estrogen patch is available under the brand name of Estraderm and comes in 2 strengths: Estraderm 100 and Estraderm 50.

The smaller doses in the estrogen patches, for example, Estraderm 50, are most unlikely to cause weight gain. Generally speaking it is possible, by juggling and/or reducing the doses of estrogen and progesterone in your hormone replacement therapy, to avoid any significant weight gain.

If, despite all these measures, hormone replacement therapy still causes unwanted weight gain, you may decide to give it up altogether, but check with your doctor first as you may be losing the great advantages that estrogen replacement therapy has for your skeleton and blood vessels. If after all consideration you decide to give up hormone replacement therapy, I suggest you consume a diet that is high in calcium, vitamin D and natural food sources of estrogen. Natural plant estrogens can be found in many foods such as green beans and soybeans. For full details of foods high in natural plant estrogens, see page 81. Good food sources of vitamin D are eggs, milk, fatty fish (tuna, salmon, sardines, herrings), fish and animal livers. Vitamin D is also produced in the skin from the energy of the sun's ultraviolet rays, so 20 to

30 minutes of sun exposure daily is a good idea, but please avoid the hottest time of the day between 10 A.M. and 3 P.M. For those who do not like vitamin D containing foods or the sun, it is a good idea to take a vitamin D supplement of 400 I.U.s daily. Vitamin D is essential to keep your bones healthy and strong during menopause and the years thereafter.

To find foods that are high in calcium, see our calcium table on page 244.

Other hormonal drugs that can cause unwanted weight gain are the oral contraceptive pill (especially high-dose formulas) that contain synthetic masculine-type progesterones. Ask your doctor for one of the newer low-dose oral contraceptive pills containing friendly, feminine progesterones. These have far less tendency to stack on extra pounds.

Women taking anabolic steroids for competitive sport and athletics gain both muscle and fat, whereas the hormone cortisone used in a variety of medical diseases causes an accumulation of fat in the face, back of the neck and abdomen. This can be offset by exercise and usually disappears once the medication is discontinued.

By going back to diagram 2, you can see that hormones act as powerful keys on our cells and greatly influence the chemical processes within the cells. Thus the type and amount of any hormonal replacement or drugs that you are taking, especially on a long-term basis, must be carefully chosen and reviewed regularly by your doctor.

4. THE WRONG DIET FOR YOUR BODY SHAPE. If four women, each one being a different body shape or type— namely gynecoid, android, thyroid or lymphatic—follow the same calorie-restricted diet, then they will lose weight at different rates and from different parts of their bodies. This is an important new discovery that makes a tailor-made diet, or, better said, an eating plan, for each of the four body

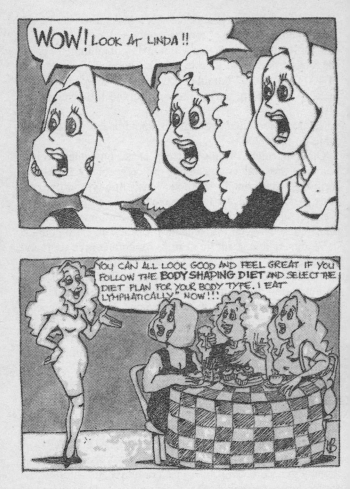

shapes essential if weight loss is to be achieved efficiently and from the desired places.

No one diet will work properly for all women, and I have

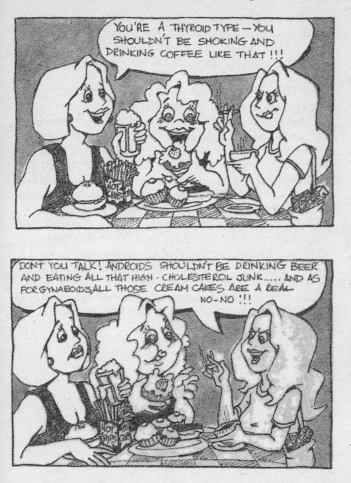

seen this time and time again. For example, if a gynecoid-shaped woman follows the eating plan for a thyroid-shaped woman, she will lose weight in the face and breasts, but not from the areas she has unwanted fat—namely her buttocks and thighs. Thus, despite restricting her calories she will retain a large bottom and thighs because she is not eating the types of foods to stimulate the inner chemical processes of her fat cells.

Similarly, if an android woman follows the eating plan for a lymphatic-shaped woman she will lose weight slowly from her legs and arms, but not from the areas where she is prone to obesity—namely her neck, trunk and abdomen.

Once again, by going back to our lonely little fat cell in diagram 2, we can see that it is vital to surround the cell with the correct balance of raw materials—hormones, nutrients, vitamins and minerals—if we are going to achieve efficient chemical processes or metabolism within the cell.

The Body-Shaping Diet will match your dominant hormonal character and body shape with the correct balance of fat, protein, carbohydrate, vitamins, minerals and water. The Body-Shaping Diet recipes are easy to follow and we explain the way they work on your metabolism. We will also include specific nutritional, naturopathic and herbal supplements to stimulate metabolism and aid weight loss for each of the four body shapes.

CHAPTER THREE

How Is Your Present Weight?

Simply by looking in the mirror it can be difficult to judge just how overweight or underweight you are. Perhaps you would prefer not to know! For those of us who would like to know, the table on the next page shows us if we fall into the desirable or normal weight range for our height and frame size.

Another more graphic way of illustrating your weight can be done by plotting your weight (along the vertical axis), alongside your height (along the horizontal axis) on the weight for height graph (see diagram 5).

If you fall into the obese range of the graph you may be subject to the following medical risks:

1. High blood pressure and cardiovascular disease
2. Diabetes
3. Respiratory problems
4. Gallstones
5. Complicated pregnancies
6. Arthritis
7. Increased risk of cancer of the breast, uterus, gallbladder and bowel

DESIRABLE WEIGHT, AGE 25 YEARS AND OVER

Height	Small Frame	Medium Frame	Large Frame
ft	lbs	lbs	lbs
4'8"	92–98	96–107	104–119
4'9"	94–101	98–110	106–122
4'10"	96–104	101–113	109–125
4'11"	99–107	104–116	112–128
5'0"	102–110	107–119	115–131
5'1"	105–113	110–122	118–132
5'2"	108–116	113–126	121–138
5'3"	111–119	116–130	125–142
5'4"	114–123	120–135	129–146
5'5"	118–127	124–139	133–150
5'6"	121–131	128–143	139–154
5'7"	126–135	132–147	141–158
5'8"	130–140	136–151	145–163
5'9"	134–144	140–155	149–168
5'10"	138–148	144–159	153–173

Note: For ages between 18 and 25 years, subtract one pound for each year under 25 years of age.

8. Hormonal and gynecological disorders such as fibroids and heavy painful periods. Obesity will cause a women to make more estrogen in her fatty tissues, which stimulates the growth of fibroids. This may also worsen endometriosis and increase menstrual blood flow and pain. As women get fatter, their level of the male hormone testosterone increases, which will increase the tendency to facial hair, greasy skin and acne.

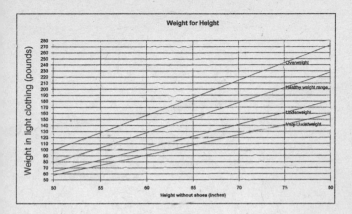

Diagram 5

Weight loss will correct these hormonal imbalances and consequently improve gynecological and skin problems.

9. Sleep apnea, the medical term for failure to breathe during sleep. This affects the hypothalamus and reduces oxygen supply to the cells, which reduces the metabolic rate and makes it much harder for you to lose weight. Sleep apnea in obese persons can have severe effects, causing a reduction in overall hormone production and a big reduction in the amount of growth hormone produced by the pituitary gland. These effects may increase the rate at which the body ages.

10. A shorter life span and higher risk of death.

If you fall into the overweight range on the graph, you will also be subject to the above ten medical risks but with less susceptibility than those in the obese range.

If you fall into the very underweight range on the graph,

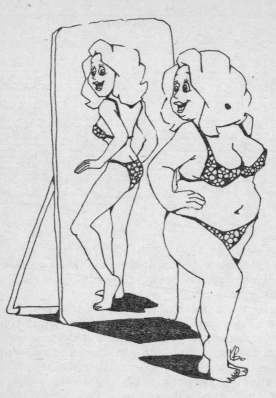

you should try to gain weight by increasing your consumption of calories and protein foods to increase fat and muscle tissue. Try to eat more bread, cereals, grains, nuts, whole wheat cakes, honey, full-fat dairy products, eggs, chicken, seafood and lean meats.

If you remain very underweight, you will be at an increased risk of the following disorders:

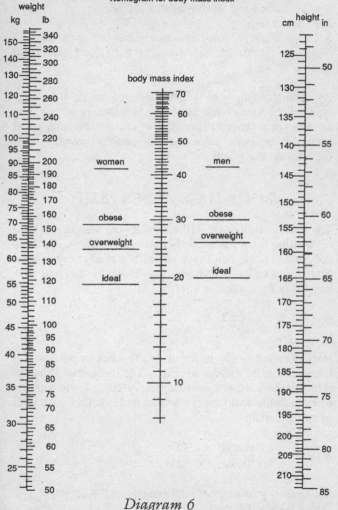

Diagram 6

1. Low levels of estrogen with an associated higher risk of osteoporosis and cardiovascular disease
2. Reduced fertility
3. Complicated pregnancies with a higher risk of intrauterine growth retardation (underweight baby) and premature labor

By understanding your weight-for-height ratio, your body type and the factors that determine your metabolic rate, you are now in a powerful position to change the things that prevent you from achieving the healthy weight range depicted on our graph.

BODY MASS INDEX (BMI)

The most scientific way of looking at your weight is a ratio or equation known as the body mass index (BMI). For those not good at math, don't tune out, as it is really very simple! You can calculate your body mass index by dividing your weight by the square of your height:

$$\text{BMI} = \frac{\text{WEIGHT}}{\text{HEIGHT} \times \text{HEIGHT}}$$

BMI is calculated in metric units. To convert pounds into kilograms, multiply your weight by 0.4536. To change inches into meters, multiply your height by 0.0254. Here is the formula to use to do the conversion and calculate your BMI in one equation:

$$\text{BMI} = \frac{\text{pounds} \times 0.4536}{(\text{inches} \quad 0.0254)^2}$$

Let's say if you weighed 150 pounds and your height is 5 feet, 8 inches (68 inches).

$$\text{Your } \mathbf{BMI} = \frac{150 \text{ pounds} \times 0.4536}{(68 \quad 0.0254)^2}$$

$$= \frac{68.04}{(1.727)^2} = \frac{68.04}{2.98}$$

$$=\quad 22.8, \text{ which falls into the healthy range}$$

of 19 to 25. In other words, you are not too heavy for your height.

If you don't like equations, you can easily work out your BMI from the scale on page 40. To use it, place a ruler between your weight (undressed) and your height (without shoes). Then read your BMI on the middle scale.

- If you are a woman you should aim to keep your BMI between 19 and 25 depending upon your build: for men BMI should fall in the range of 20 to 26. By keeping your BMI in these ranges you will enjoy better general health.
- Overweight is considered between the upper limit of normal body mass index (25 for women) and a body mass index of 29.
- Obesity is defined as a body mass index greater than 29.
- Anorexia nervosa (see page 295) is associated with a body mass index of less than 17.

When weighing yourself choose the *same time* of the day, wearing no clothes. Weight can vary by 2 to 4 pounds over one day due to fluid retention, constipation, a full bladder, exercise, hormonal changes, time of the menstrual cycle and other factors. Thus, weighing yourself once or twice a week is sufficient, less frustrating and less prone to small errors.

THE BODY-SHAPING
EATING PLAN STRATEGY

The body-shaping eating plan consists of two simple steps:

1) STEP ONE
TO LOSE WEIGHT. This is desirable if your body mass index is over 25. You can use the Body-Shaping Diet menus, found between pages 104 and 136, to bring your weight back down into the ideal body mass index range of 19 to 25.

2) STEP TWO
TO MAINTAIN IDEAL BODY WEIGHT. Once you have achieved a weight and body shape that please you it is important that you do not discard the Body-Shaping Diet. At this stage, ideally, your weight will fall into the body mass index range of 19 to 25. To maintain your desired weight and figure, follow the Body-Shaping Diet menus found between pages 137 and 157 and practice the body-shaping exercises beginning on page 281.

CHAPTER FOUR

THE ANDROID-SHAPED WOMAN

The classical android-shaped woman is rather square shaped with a solid big-boned frame, giving her a powerful and athletic appearance. Her dominant gland is the adrenal gland, of which there are two situated on top of each kidney. These two small fleshy glands produce the powerful hormones cortisone and adrenaline as well as a variety of male hormones (androgens). The android woman will have a tendency to overproduce male hormones, particularly if she becomes obese. These male hormones will make her look more masculine and may stimulate the growth of facial and body hair, greasy skin and acne.

The powerful adrenal hormones make her energetic and strong with good staying power when others around her need a coffee break or sugar fix. Android-shaped women are usually not sugarholics or sweet tooths, but instead crave foods high in cholesterol and salt that act to stimulate their dominant adrenal glands to pump out more steroid hormones, such as cortisone and androgens. These hormones are anabolic, meaning that they promote an increase in body muscle and fat that accumulates around the jowls, neck, shoulders, upper arms, trunk and abdomen. This further exaggerates the tendency toward a masculine appearance.

If android women become overweight, the excess fat is deposited in the upper half of the body, i.e., above the hips, and we call this upper-level body obesity, which contrasts with the lower-level body obesity typical of gynecoid-shaped women. Android or upper-level body obesity is more dangerous for health than lower-level body obesity, as it is associated with a higher level of the medical complications of obesity such as cardiovascular disease, high blood pressure, high cholesterol and diabetes, which may shorten life span.

Thus, it is important to encourage android-shaped women to maintain their body weight within the normal range for their height or more specifically to maintain their body mass index (see page 41) in the normal range of 19–25 kg/m².

Body fat is a significant source of production of the sex hormones estrogen and androgens (male hormones). As the amount of fat in the body increases, so will the amount of estrogen and androgens produced in the fat increase. Conversely, weight loss and a reduction in body fat is associated with a lowering in the levels of estrogen and androgens. Thus, it is easy to understand how hormonal imbalances can be corrected by weight normalization.

The Body-Shaping Diet for android-shaped women (see page 104) is scientifically designed to help weight loss and hormonal imbalance in two ways:

1. It is low in cholesterol, saturated fat and salt, which will reduce the excessive production of androgens from the adrenal glands.
2. It promotes weight loss in the upper part of the body and abdomen, which further lowers body androgen levels.

All women produce both male and female hormones in their ovaries, adrenal glands and fat. Indeed, women chemically convert male hormones into female hormones and if a woman does not produce male hormones, she will not make any estrogen. If the levels of androgens are excessive compared to the levels of the female hormone estrogen, the body shape becomes more masculine and acne may occur. What we are aiming to achieve with the Body-Shaping Diet is a rebalancing of the levels of female and male hormones (androgens). Reducing male hormone levels and upper-body fat causes the appearance and body physique to become more feminine.

POLYCYSTIC OVARY SYNDROME

At this point it is worthwhile mentioning a rather common hormonal disorder that is more likely to occur in android-shaped women, especially if they become overweight. This is called the polycystic ovary syndrome, and in this disorder the ovary looks different from a normal ovary (see diagram 7). In a normal ovary, the eggs or follicles are distributed evenly throughout the ovary whereas in the polycystic ovary, follicles varying in size from 2 to 8 millimeters are lined up around the edge of the ovary. The polycystic ovary does not function in an ideal way: It usually produces excessive amounts of male hormones and does not produce a regular supply of fertile eggs. Thus the menstrual cycle is usually irregular and most commonly menstrual bleeding is infrequent, occurring only two or three times per year.

Obesity may trigger the polycystic ovary syndrome and will cause it to be more pronounced. In obese women the large deposits of fat produce excessive male hormones, which act on the polycystic ovary and stimulate it to produce even more male hormones.

Thus, in obese android women with polycystic ovary syndrome we have three sources of production of excessive male hormones: the fat, the adrenal glands and the ovaries. Little wonder that many of these women complain of acne and excess facial and body hair. If the level of male hormones

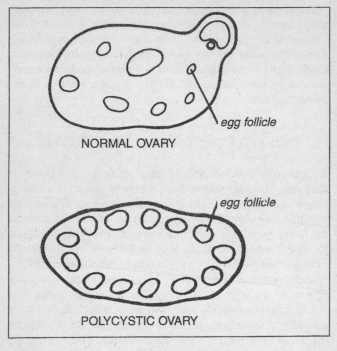

NORMAL OVARY

egg follicle

egg follicle

POLYCYSTIC OVARY

Diagram 7

becomes very high, loss of scalp hair may occur, with the hair thinning in the frontal and temporal areas of the scalp.

Mild cases of polycystic ovary syndrome can often be corrected simply by losing excess weight, and women with polycystic ovaries should keep their body mass index around 21 kilogram/m². Ideal weight equals height² × 21 (reference: *Women's Hormone Problems*, Dr. John Eden, First Edition 1991). Thus if you are 170 cm (5′7″) in height your ideal body weight = 1.7 meters × 1.7 meters × 21 = 60.69, or approximately 61 kg (134 lbs).

Once ideal weight is achieved, regular menstrual bleeding often resumes and male hormone levels reduce, with a resultant decrease in acne and facial hair. More severe or resistant cases of polycystic ovary syndrome will require the use of specific hormone therapy designed to block the effect of the excess male hormones and produce a regular menstrual cycle. This tailor-made hormone therapy will cure acne and greatly reduce facial hair. Hormonal therapy that will help these problems are an estrogenic contraceptive pill or the tablet called Aldactone. See your own doctor about these treatments.

In android-shaped women with very high levels of male hormones, weight loss can be easier and more effective if the excess of male hormones is corrected first, which can be done with hormone therapy. Suitable drugs to reduce male hormones are an estrogenic contraceptive pill or Aldactone.

BEVERLY'S CASE HISTORY

Beverly was a very mature woman for twenty-five and exuded an air of relaxed confidence and power that enabled her to run a large furniture factory successfully. She had been struggling with excess body and facial hair for seven years ever since she had started to gain weight at the age of eighteen. In typical android style, her weight gain was mostly in the upper part of her body around her face, neck, chest and abdomen. Her excessive weight and facial hair, combined with her android shape, gave Beverly a somewhat masculine appearance.

Beverly's periods had started late, when she was seventeen, and had always been infrequent so I thought it highly likely that she had the polycystic ovary syndrome.

Beverly requested a cure for her excess hairiness and

assistance in losing weight. She was about to start a new relationship and wanted to look and feel more feminine. She was also contemplating having children in her late twenties.

Beverly's blood test revealed excessive levels of male hormones and raised cholesterol. An ultrasound scan of her pelvic area showed polycystic ovaries.

Beverly weighed 172 pounds, her height was 5'5" and her body mass index was between 28 and 29. Her blood pressure was higher than normal and she had excessive hair around her chin, upper lip, navel and nipples and very hairy arms and legs.

Beverly was a classic android-shaped woman with the added hormone imbalance of polycystic ovary syndrome. She craved fatty and salty foods such as pizza, salami, ham and fish and chips. These foods were stimulating her adrenal glands to produce excessive amounts of male hormones, which had gradually increased her body hair and weight over the last seven years. Beverly was utterly amazed to learn that her beloved fish and chips could be increasing her body hair and masculinity, as she had not realized that a high-fat diet could cause a hormone imbalance. She had thought that she simply took after her father and that she was destined for shaving cream and the razor blade.

Beverly was started on the Body-Shaping Diet for android-shaped women (see page 104). The menus in this eating plan contain foods that are high in estrogenic substances that would have a feminizing effect upon her physique. See page 81 for a complete list of foods high in natural estrogens. The Body-Shaping Diet for android women contains protein that comes mainly from nonanimal sources such as grains, cereals, nuts, seeds, legumes and fish. These protein sources are high in fiber and low in saturated fat and salt and they do not stimulate the adrenal glands to produce anabolic hormones. Only small servings of chicken, lean red meats and low-fat dairy products are allowed in the Body-Shaping Diet for android women. Commercially raised hens should be avoided as they may be fed anabolic hormones to make them grow quickly; only free-range chicken should be eaten.

Liver-friendly foods such as garlic, onion, chives, dandelion, watercress, beets and carrots are included as they act as tonics for the liver. An active and healthy liver is required in android-shaped women because the liver breaks down and inactivates the steroid hormones, which tend to be present in excessive amounts.

Beverly applied her enormous enthusiasm and willpower to following the Body-Shaping Diet and was pleased to see results after only two months. She had lost 17.5 pounds in weight and had slimmed down over her upper body. Her blood pressure was now normal and her cholesterol levels were down by two points.

Beverly was anxious to have a regular menstrual period and reduce her facial hair so I recommended that she start a tailor-made oral contraceptive pill containing two different hormones. This contained the female hormone estrogen and an antimale hormone Androcur, which would block the effect of her excessive male hormones upon the hair follicles. Androcur is a potent antimale hormone, which has been proven to cure acne and greatly reduce excess facial and body hair. It is a slow-acting hormone and I explained to Beverly that Androcur would take a full twelve months to fully exert its effect in controlling body hair. Androcur is presently unavailable in the United States, but is available in Canada, Europe, the United Kingdom, South Africa and Australia.

Well, after twelve months one could hardly recognize Beverly as the same person who had originally presented to me looking overweight, hairy and masculine. She now weighed 126 pounds, which for a height of 5'5" put her body mass index at 21, ideal for a woman with polycystic ovary syndrome.

She no longer looked obese and solidly square in shape

and indeed looked slim and decidedly feminine. Her facial features looked finer as did her neck and muscular limbs. Her previously large pendulous breasts and protruding abdomen were no longer obvious as she had lost large amounts of weight from these areas.

Beverly was very happy in her relationship and said that for the first time in many years she now felt like a woman and loved looking feminine. She assured me that she intended to remain that way and would stick to the Body-Shaping Diet and exercise program for the rest of her life.

FRIEDA'S CASE HISTORY

Frieda came from a Germanic background and had inherited the stocky android frame of her grandmother. She had worked hard with her husband on their large property growing grains and raising cattle for thirty years and had recently moved to the city. She was forty-nine and just beginning menopause, and wanted to avoid middle-aged spread. With this aim in mind she avoided sweets and cakes but continued to enjoy a diet high in meats, cheese and salty foods. Frieda was having trouble maintaining her body weight and had started accumulating fat around her neck, upper arms and abdomen, which was not surprising due to her adoption of a more sedentary lifestyle and her high-fat diet. She complained to me that her appearance was becoming more masculine and that she noticed increasing amounts of hair growing on her face.

On examination, Frieda weighed 168 pounds, which for her height of 5′3″ put her body mass index between 29 and 30. Her blood pressure was slightly raised and blood tests revealed very low levels of the female hormone estrogen, in keeping with her menopausal state, and normal levels of male hormones. Frieda's increasing facial hair was due to the fact that now she was menopausal her hormonal balanc had changed and she had relatively more male hormones than female hormones. Her ovaries were no longer producing significant amounts of hormones and her supplies of male hormones were coming from her increasing fat supplies and her adrenal glands.

Thus, I explained to Frieda that if we were to reduce her levels of male hormones we would need to change her diet so that her body fat reduced and her adrenal glands were not overstimulated. The perfect diet for this aim, and the one that also matched her body shape, was the Body-Shaping Diet for android women. This diet was a slight cultural shock for Frieda, whose Central European family had always thought that red meats, eggs, dairy products and salty foods were the foundation of a strong, healthy body.

Still, we agreed it is never too late to change one's way of thinking and Frieda decided to try the recipes and menus in the Body-Shaping Diet for android women. She began eating far more raw fruits and vegetables, grains, legumes, seeds, nuts and fish than she ever had and gradually began to taste the more subtle flavors of food, as her meals were no longer seasoned with salt. Initially, she really missed her fried foods, especially her Vienna schnitzel, but as she began to notice her body shape changing her satisfaction and pleasure made it easier to resist these high-fat foods.

Six months after her first visit, Frieda was no longer craving salt and fried foods and told me that her favorite food was now vegetable and mixed bean soup. She felt that she had formed an entirely new set of taste buds on her tongue. Frieda had lost 28 pounds and now weighed 140 pounds, which for her height of 5′3″ put her body mass index just under 25. She looked far more feminine, as her neck and shoulders had slimmed down and her abdomen was now flat and muscular. This was due to the combination of the Body-Shaping Diet for android-shaped women and the body-shaping exercise program, which had also brought her blood pressure back to normal and increased her fitness.

Frieda felt so good about her new self that she now wanted to start hormone replacement therapy to eliminate her facial hair and stop hot flushes. I started her on a combination of natural estrogen and a small dose of the antimale hormone Androcur, which would stop the male hormones from stimulating her facial hair follicles.

Twelve months later Frieda looked fit, trim and feminine and her facial hair was greatly diminished. She was content to stay on the Body-Shaping Diet for her shape indefinitely, with a few special treats thrown in at birthdays and holiday times.

MAGGIE'S CASE HISTORY

Maggie had traveled a long distance from one of Australia's country towns to consult me about her rapid gain in weight of 44 pounds in just over two years. She had gone from 134 pounds to 178 pounds, which for her body height of 5'3" gave her a body mass index of just over 31.

She was confused, depressed and totally bewildered because she had gained this weight despite the fact that she had not changed her eating habits in twenty years. Her increasing weight made her very unfit and she was breathless as she sat down in front of me after climbing the flight of stairs to my office. Maggie had come to see me because none of the doctors she had consulted would believe that she was not a closet eater.

Maggie told me that her problem had started just over two years ago when she had been put on hormone tablets to control her menopausal hot flushes. After this her weight began to soar and because she was an android shape she had accumulated fat in the upper part of her body. She had developed a fat face and neck, big arms, a thick trunk and a big protruding abdomen, which she tried to conceal under a loose-fitting caftan dress. Her diet had not changed; she had always been a big meat eater and was not partial to sweets or chocolates. Maggie was also battling with high cholesterol and raised blood pressure, which had not been helped by her hormone tablets.

I explained to Maggie that android-shaped women such as herself tended to gain weight easily and that hormone replacement therapy could aggravate this tendency. She had had a hysterectomy and therefore did not require the hormone progesterone, which had been given to her in the form of a large dose of Provera. Synthetic progesterones often have an anabolic action—in other words, they tend to promote an increase in body fat and fluids. Thus, the first step was to stop her progesterone tablets.

Estrogen tablets are more likely to promote weight gain than are the nonoral forms of estrogen such as the estrogen patch, so I switched Maggie to an estrogen patch and stopped her estrogen tablets. To reduce her fatigue I prescribed evening primrose oil 2000 mg daily, vitamin B complex and calcium and magnesium supplements.

Maggie was started on the Body-Shaping Diet for android women (see page 97) and I also asked her to avoid salt and drink ten glasses of water daily. She was greatly relieved that a doctor had finally believed her and taken her story seriously as up until then she admitted to me that she seriously thought she was going mad.

Six months later she returned having lost all the excess 44 pounds she had gained after starting hormone replacement therapy. She was back to her 134 pounds, had returned to playing tennis and looked years younger than when I had seen her six months ago.

Maggie had encouraged several of her overweight menopausal friends to follow the Body-Shaping Diet for their particular body shape and all had achieved a successful outcome. She had always been a great cook and popular hostess and was now thinking of setting up a restaurant serving menus from the Body-Shaping Diet book in her town.

CHAPTER FIVE

THE GYNECOID-SHAPED WOMAN

The gynecoid shape is a common female body shape. This type of woman is pear-shaped, with average- to small-sized shoulders, variably sized breasts, a small waist and curvaceous buttocks and rounded thighs. She is the voluptuous Marilyn Monroe type and was typically the subject of the great French impressionist painters. She is the model of yesterday and is generally more cuddly and curvy than the lean to skinny models of today.

The female hormone estrogen produced by the sex glands or ovaries causes the selective deposition of fat cells in the areas of the breasts, buttocks and thighs. The gynecoid woman usually has plentiful supplies of estrogen if her ovaries are healthy and indeed if she becomes overweight, she often has excessive amounts of estrogen or a hyperestrogenic state. Excessive weight will be deposited particularly in the lower half of the body in the feminine areas such as buttocks, pelvis, hips, thighs and eventually the breasts. It is unfortunate that this type of fatty tissue may become uneven and lumpy, resulting in tenacious cellulite. We call this type of obesity lower-segment body obesity as it is mainly confined below the waist. The large deposits of fatty tissue are in themselves hormonally active and produce significant amounts of the sex hormone estrogen, in addition to the ovaries pumping out their own monthly surges of estrogen. It is thus easy to understand why an overweight gynecoid-shaped woman tends to have high levels of estrogen, which will act to further exaggerate the deposition of fat cells in the feminine curvy areas, especially the buttocks and thighs. Thus the gynecoid woman is often frustrated by her large bottom or rear, which may start to droop posterially as she ages. Elizabeth Taylor is a classical gynecoid woman who has not always managed to keep her estrogenic curves under control.

The dominant hormonal glands in the gynecoid woman are the ovaries and if you are a gynecoid woman, as a generalization, you will normally be fertile and become pregnant easily!

Many gynecoid women find that when they become significantly overweight they develop health problems due to excessive estrogen production from their ovaries and fat deposits. There are several organs in the body that are very receptive or sensitive to the effects of the hormone estrogen, especially the breasts and uterus. Estrogen stimulates the breasts and uterus to enlarge and if excessive levels of estrogen are sustained, the breasts may become larger, tender and lumpy and the uterus congested. This latter effect can result in increasingly heavy menstrual bleeding, menstrual cramps and increase the risk of fibroids and endometriosis.

You can now understand how obesity increases the incidence of gynecological problems in women. We also know that obese women have a higher incidence of cancer of the uterus and breasts, partly because of the link between excess weight, hormone imbalance and body organ sensitivity. Gynecoid women, and indeed all women, can reduce their risk of cancer by avoiding obesity—another very good reason to follow the Body-Shaping Diet.

CHARLOTTE'S CASE HISTORY

My patient Charlotte came to see me in a desperate state. She was obsessed with the appearance of her rather large bottom, which drooped down the back of her thighs. Moreover, Charlotte's bottom was covered with stretch marks, a testimony to the rapid and repetitive weight cycling she had experienced over the last decade. Charlotte was an example of why fast weight-loss diets don't work, as they had decreased her muscle mass (lean body tissue) and thus after each crash diet she found she could tolerate less calories than before. Because she could not stick to such a restrictive diet forever, within a few months of stopping her diet all her weight loss plus a few extra pounds would come back. Poor Charlotte had experienced this weight cycling at least a dozen times and was extremely depressed and unmotivated. I told Charlotte that any diet that promises rapid weight loss would end up making her fatter in the long term and this was why her bottom and upper thighs had slowly increased over the years.

Charlotte was a typical gynecoid woman, very much influenced by the monthly fluctuations of her sex hormones, and she found that she gained around 4.4 pounds before every menstrual period. Premenstrually her food cravings became worse and she binged on creamy foods and sugary quick fixes to cheer and comfort herself. I explained to Charlotte that sugar really becomes a problem when it is consumed in large doses or if it is combined with creamy, fatty foods, such as in the cream buns and layer cakes she wolfed down before her period.

Charlotte had thought that she was jinxed or terribly unlucky as on each of her crash diets she had lost weight first from her face, neck, breasts and abdomen, with her bottom and thighs remaining amazingly the same and full of pouchy cellulite. She was quite angry that no one had ever explained the relationship of body shape to hormona imbalance and weight excess, as it all seemed so logical to her now. However, I explained it was a new scientific discovery.

Charlotte was eating high-calorie refined creamy foods that were stimulating her dominant ovaries to pump out more estrogen. These foods also caused fat deposition around the lower half of her body and this fatty tissue produced even more estrogen. Her high levels of estrogen caused fat to be laid down around her buttocks and thighs, perpetuating her matronly derriere. Poor Charlotte was well down the road to becoming a middle-aged blimp and was frightened she would become like her gynecoid-shaped mother who had ended up 187 pounds and 5'3" at the age of fifty-five.

Now that Charlotte understood the link between her gynecoid shape, hormonal imbalance, and weight problem she was ready to stick to an eating plan that could bring these three factors into harmony. She realized that her binges of creamy and sugary foods were not only making her fat but also causing fatigue and slowly eroding her health. She was finally craving good health and well-being more than she was craving fat and refined sugar. Charlotte was now ready to begin and stick to the Body-Shaping Diet designed for the gynecoid woman (see page 112).

At this point Charlotte weighed 150 pounds at a height of 5'2", putting her body mass index at just over 27. I explained to Charlotte that she must avoid the saturated fats found in full-fat dairy products, fried foods, creamy foods, processed foods and take-out food. Alcohol was also on the forbidden list, as it is very high in calories and contains natural estrogens, which in Charlotte's case were plentiful enough.

Charlotte went off armed with the Body-Shaping Diet and an appointment to see me in six weeks. When she returned she bounced into my office looking energetic and I noted the big improvement in her complexion. She was delighted with her loss of 7 pounds because for the first time in her

life she had lost it from her bottom and thighs. She remarked
that, although the rate of weight loss was slower than with
her previous crash diets, she was finding it so easy as she
was not tired and really enjoyed the nutritious foods in the
Body-Shaping Diet. Her cravings for junk food had gone
and she felt more inclined to exercise regularly. I told her
to stick to the diet for the gynecoid woman and return in
eight weeks.

Next time I saw Charlotte she had lost another 9 pounds.
She was wearing a close-fitting pair of denim jeans and
looked slinky and attractive. She was doing it for herself
and was more confident; the confidence came from inside
Charlotte as she could see that the cellulite was disappearing
from her bottom and thighs and the shape of her body was
changing in a way she had always desired.

Twelve months after starting the Body-Shaping Diet,
Charlotte weighed 115 pounds and could fit into a size ten
pair of jeans. She was still a gynecoid-shaped woman, but
her fat cells had redistributed themselves more evenly
throughout her body and were no longer all concentrated in
her bottom and thighs. Charlotte liked herself and what's
more she liked the feeling of being in control of her body.

CHRISTINE'S CASE HISTORY

Christine, aged thirty-two, had been married for three years
and was feeling most dejected by her inability to become
pregnant due to the condition of endometriosis. Endometriosis is the gynecological disorder that occurs when the lining
of the uterus (endometrium) grows outward through the
fallopian tubes and spills into the pelvic and abdominal
cavities where it grows much like a weed. Every month
when menstruation occurs this abnormally sited endometrium bleeds into the pelvic cavity, causing painful periods
and scarring of the internal organs. Christine had been treated

for six months with a powerful drug called Danazol, which is masculine in its effect and blocks the action of the female hormone estrogen in the body. Unfortunately, when the Danazol was discontinued, her endometriosis, once again under the influence of estrogen, had started to regrow, causing abdominal and pelvic pains.

Christine was a classical gynecoid-shaped woman with large curvaceous buttocks and rounded thighs that touched together and were dimpled with cellulite. She had gained 26 pounds since being married and now weighed 154 pounds at a height of 5'4", which put her body mass index between 26 and 27. This weight gain was due to her change in lifestyle after being married, when she stopped exercising and began cooking fried and creamy foods to delight her husband. They also drank two or three glasses of wine with each evening meal, adding around 250 calories to the meal.

Christine did not want to go back on Danazol as she believed it had contributed to her weight gain and she had come to see me searching for a more natural approach to her obesity and endometriosis. I explained to her that her high-fat, high-calorie diet and excessive weight had caused high levels of estrogen in her body, which had stimulated the growth of the endometriosis. If she were to follow the Body-Shaping Diet for the gynecoid-shaped woman, she would gradually slim down, resulting in lower levels of estrogen and shrinkage of the deposits of endometriosis in her pelvis.

She was most interested to learn that a high-fat diet also caused an increased production of inflammatory chemicals in the body known as prostaglandins. These excessive prostaglandins caused increased inflammation in her uterus and tubes, thus increasing her pelvic pain and congestion.

To reduce inflammation and congestion, I prescribed evening primrose oil 3000 mg daily, calcium 600 mg daily, vitamin E 1000 I.U. daily, vitamin C with bioflavonoids 2000 mg daily and beta-carotene 10 mg daily. These nutritional supplements would be slower to act than Danazol as they did not directly block the production of the body's estrogen, but rather strengthened the immune system, which would gradually control the endometriosis.

I sent Christine off armed with the Body-Shaping Diet for the gynecoid-shaped woman (see page 112), the prescription for nutritional supplements and the body-shaping exercise program. This exercise program would not only reduce her excessive buttocks and thighs, but also improve circulation to the pelvic organs, which is a vital strategy for all women battling with endometriosis.

Christine returned after three months reporting that her pelvic pain and menstrual periods were much better. However, she had lost only 7 pounds in weight and none from her buttocks and thighs. On further questioning, I discovered that Christine had been doing only two out of the three things I had prescribed. She was taking her nutritional supplements and exercising, but when it came to the Body-Shaping Diet she was following her own variation. Due to pressures from her husband, she was still eating too much fat and creamy foods and found it difficult to cook two meals, one for herself and one for her husband. I suggested that she cajole her husband into sticking to the Body-Shaping Diet with her, with the added reward that by reducing to her normal body weight she would increase her chances of becoming pregnant and having a trouble-free pregnancy. I reinforced that unless she stuck carefully to the Body-Shaping Diet for her gynecoid shape, she would find it very difficult to lose weight from her buttocks and thighs.

Well, this trick really worked and I did not hear from Christine for another year. She popped into the waiting room one day in the full bloom of pregnancy and began enthusiastically telling all the waiting patients that the Body-Shaping Diet was a surefire way to become pregnant. I didn't design the Body-Shaping Diet to increase fertility; its primary aim is to reshape and normalize body weight, bu it is fascinating to discover time and time again that by correcting the diet we not only slim down but rebalance our hormones and achieve a superior quality of life.

By the way, I forgot to mention that Christine did lose weight from her buttocks and thighs but became pregnant before the process was complete. The Body-Shaping Diet should not be followed during pregnancy or breastfeeding, but Christine told me that she would resume it after breastfeeding as she had never felt better than when she was on it.

REBECCA'S CASE HISTORY

Menstrual cramps are a common problem for many women and few realize that they can be related to poor diet, obesity or lack of fitness. This was so for Rebecca, a classic gynecoid-shaped woman, who weighed 168 pounds at a height of 5'1", giving her a body mass index of 31. Most of her obesity was in the breasts, buttocks and upper thighs associated with well-advanced cellulite. Rebecca's blood test revealed high levels of estrogen and a tendency toward diabetes (prediabetic state). Her uterus was moderately enlarged and congested and tilted backward (retroverted).

Rebecca was only twenty-three but she had been overweight for eight years, ever since leaving school and ceasing regular sports. She desperately wanted to lose her large drooping bottom and thick thighs and she was getting nowhere with her severe incapacitating menstrual cramps that lasted for two days out of every month. She took large doses of Ponstel, which dulled the pain, but every month the bleeding seemed to be getting heavier and more painful.

I felt fortunate to be able to assess Rebecca at the young age of twenty-three, as I might otherwise have seen her at age forty, diabetic, very overweight and with an enlarged fibroid uterus or possibly a hysterectomy. As I explained my prognosis to Rebecca, we both realized that she needed to start and stick to a lifetime plan. If Rebecca was going to change her pear shape and eradicate cellulite from her buttocks and thighs, she would need to stick to the Body-Shaping Diet for the gynecoid woman for most of her life. I explained to Rebecca that although the Body-Shaping Diet could be used to achieve a so-called classically beautiful figure, this was not the aim for all women and indeed not necessary for happiness or high self-esteem. In her case, I felt it was more important that she lose around 40 pounds to bring her body mass index into the normal range of 19 to 25, which would give her a weight of around 128 pounds for a height of 5'1". This would reduce her high estrogen levels, greatly reduce her period problems and reverse her prediabetic tendency. After these things had been achieved with the Body-Shaping Diet, she could then slim down her bottom and thighs further if this was important for her self-esteem.

To prevent menstrual cramps, I advised a course of nutritional supplements, namely iron amino acid chelate 100 mg, calcium 800 mg, magnesium 600 mg, evening primrose oil 3000 mg and an antioxidant formula containing vitamin C 2000 mg, vitamin E 500 I.U., beta-carotene 10 mg. I find this a useful program for many women wanting to reduce menstrual cramps and bleeding by natural means. We decided against the oral contraceptive pill as a treatment for period pains as the synthetic hormones it contained could possibly aggravate her cellulite. For many women, however, the oral contraceptive pill is an excellent way to prevent painful periods.

Rebecca went off keen to begin the Body-Shaping Diet for her gynecoid shape and body-shaping exercise program and promised to return in three months. When she did, her story was most inspiring as she had a significant reduction in her cellulite, had lost 18 pounds and had been able to cope without the usual megadoses of Ponstel.

One year after our first encounter, Rebecca had achieved her goals and the thing she found surprising was the simplicity and easiness of the Body-Shaping Diet. In contrast to other diets she had tried, the Body-Shaping Diet did not make her tired, hungry and miserable and she enjoyed inviting friends over to share her meals. She now looked great in a bikini and was free of cellulite at a weight of 123 pounds. From my point of view, I was interested to note that her uterus was no longer enlarged and her blood estrogen and sugar levels were now normal.

THE LYMPHATIC-SHAPED WOMAN

In the lymphatic-shaped woman, fat is generally distributed evenly all over the body. The head and face are round in shape, the neck is short and the limbs are rather thick and straight up and down. The lymphatic-shaped woman appears more overweight than she really is, due to fluid retention in the fatty layers of the body. This may give a rather pudgy or swollen look to the feet, ankles, hands and wrists.

Fluid retention occurs because the return of blood through the veins in the arms and legs back to the heart is sluggish due to weak valves within the veins and poor muscle tone in the limbs. Fluid also tends to accumulate in the subcutaneous tissues between the skin and the muscle layer because of an inefficient lymphatic system.

The lymphatic system comprises a network of small tubes or vessels that collect subcutaneous fluids and return them to the blood circulation via the thoracic duct (see diagram on page 67). These lymphatic vessels pass through lymph glands in the groin, abdomen and armpits where the fluid is filtered and cleansed before emptying into the circulation. In lymphatic-shaped women, the subcutaneous lymphatic vessels may be deficient in number and quality and may become enlarged and congested. This predisposes to puffy, thick limbs that may contain so much excess subcutaneous fluid that on pressing them with the fingertips, a dent is left on the limbs for several minutes. This is called pitting edema by doctors. Lymphatic- type women often use diuretic drugs to try to control this retention of fluid that is such a common problem for them. Diuretic drugs stimulate the kidneys to excrete fluid and salt, which gives temporary improvement in fluid retention but does not help the underlying weakness of the veins and lymphatic vessels. Thus, the subcutaneous tissues remain spongy in nature and will swell when fluid once again accumulates in this layer.

The bones are not very obvious in the lymphatic type as they are covered by a thicker layer of fat and fluid. This contrasts with the thyroid type whose bone structure is very evident through their thinner subcutaneous layer. The thyroid woman is the bony type; the lymphatic woman is the cuddly, round type in appearance.

Because the vessels and glands of the lymphatic system tend to be inefficient, problems with the immune system may occur, as the lymphatic system forms an important part of the body's immune system. Thus problems such as swollen glands, tonsillitis, excessive mucus or allergies may occur, especially if the diet is high in dairy products or processed foods containing artificial chemicals. Excessive mucus and allergies may result in sinusitis, hay fever, sore throats, bronchitis or asthma.

Lymphatic-type women usually crave dairy products, which are not metabolized efficiently and result in weight gain and excessive mucus production in the body. To lose excessive fat and fluid lymphatic types need to follow a diet that is very low in or free of dairy products and salt (see Body-Shaping Diet for lymphatic types, page 121).

A regular exercise program is vital and the exercises in the body-shaping exercise program are designed to slim down the arms and legs by improving muscle tone and

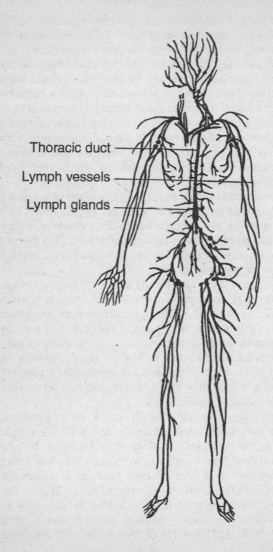

Thoracic duct

Lymph vessels

Lymph glands

increasing the return of venous blood and lymphatic fluid to the heart. Good muscle tone in the limbs is essential to aid the muscular pump that stimulates the return flow of blood and subcutaneous fluid against the force of gravity upward to the heart. Swimming, inverted yoga postures, riding an exercise bike, power walking and jogging are excellent exercise strategies for lymphatic-shaped women. These types of exercise are often followed by an increased output of urine over the next twenty-four hours, as the kidneys excrete the excessive fluid returned to the heart by the muscles in the limbs during exercise.

Many lymphatic-type women are relatively inactive or sedentary in their lifestyle and have avoided sports during childhood. Indeed they often dislike exercise and competitive sports, as unlike the thyroid types they are not quick movers and they lack the enduring physical stamina of the android types. Their personalities are often relaxed and creative so that they prefer indoor activities such as cooking, painting, reading or entertaining. So it may take some time before a lymphatic-type woman can be coaxed into a regular energetic exercise program. Unless this is achieved it is very difficult for her to slim down her legs, arms and trunk and replace spongy, subcutaneous tissue with muscle. Lymphatic types will find it difficult to tolerate occupations requiring prolonged standing or sitting in one position all day as without regular contraction of the limb muscles, fluid will quickly accumulate in the legs and feet.

Lymphatic women have a low metabolic rate and do not burn calories easily, so for them the avoidance of excessive weight is more difficult than for all the other body shapes. If a lymphatic type eats an ice cream it will be converted to fat, whereas the thyroid-type woman will burn up its contained calories far more efficiently. This is somewhat unfair and the lymphatic woman needs to stimulate her metabolic rate with regular exercise and a diet free of dairy products and low in saturated fats but high in raw fruits and vegetables.

The sluggish metabolism of the lymphatic type can be stimulated by specific foods and nutritional supplements that increase the efficiency of the intracellular biochemistry. This will start to break down excessive fat tissue and improve function of the thyroid gland. To achieve this I recommend that you regularly consume, say twice weekly, the following foods:

seaweed	sesame seeds
fresh garlic and onion,	green magna
horseradish	(barley grass
raw vegetable juices	extract)
(preferably organically grown)	dry spices such as
citrus fruits (oranges, lemons,	chili and ginger
grapefruits, limes, mandarins)	alfalfa sprouts

SPECIFIC NUTRITIONAL SUPPLEMENTS TO BOOST THE METABOLIC RATE OR LIGHT YOUR INTRACELLULAR FIRES

1. Amino acid tablets—one, twice daily
2. Trace minerals—calcium 500 mg, magnesium 100 mg, potassium 100 mg, zinc 25 mg, manganese 10 mg, chromium 250 mcg, iodine 50 mcg, molybdenum 200 mcg (daily doses)
3. Evening primrose oil 2000 mg daily
4. Ginseng root extract 500 mg daily
5. Essential blood factors—organic iron 50 mg, folic acid 300 mcg, vitamin B12 50 mcg, vitamin B6 50 mg, vitamin E 100 I.U. (daily doses). These factors are essential for cellular division, new cellular activity and healthy function of the cell's genetic material. In simple terms one

could say that they are vital factors for the genetic computer program that runs and controls each cell. Women should check with their own doctor first before taking an iron supplement as unnecessary iron can be harmful.

6. Spirulina or kelp tablets—2 daily

This particular combination of nutritional factors works together, aiding each other in a synergistic way and acting as an intracellular tonic. After taking these nutritional supplements for several months, the lymphatic-shaped woman will find it easier to lose weight while following the Body-Shaping Diet and exercise program. She will have a higher metabolic rate and find that she has more energy to give to the body-shaping exercise program.

The lymphatic-shaped woman will also benefit from foods, herbs and nutritional supplements designed to stimulate her sluggish circulation and lymphatic system. Such supplements will strengthen the weak connective tissues in her blood vessels and swollen lymphatic vessels, reducing vessel fragility. Thus, her capillaries and lymphatic channels will not be so leaky or permeable and fluid will not so readily ooze through vessel walls to accumulate in her spongy subcutaneous layer. As a result, the limbs and abdomen slim down and look less thick and congested. To achieve this effect, I recommend:

1. Vitamin C with bioflavonoids—2000 mg daily
2. Buckwheat in the form of grain, bread and porridge
3. Beta-hydroxyethyl-rutosides—500 to 1000 mg daily. This is a bioflavonoid, which is a vitamin related to vitamin C.
4. The herbs *ruscus aculeatus* (butcher's broom) 200 mg, *aesculus* (horse chestnut) 200 mg, *hamamelis* (witch hazel) 200 mg, *ranunculaceae* (pulsatilla) 25 to 50 mg. *Herbs should not be taken during pregnancy without consulting your doctor.*

5. The herbs clivers and pokeroot (phytolacca), which have astringent properties and also act as lymphatic cleansers

The lymphatic type can also reduce fluid retention by using foods and herbs that are tonics for the kidneys—in other words, they stimulate kidney function and the excretion of excess fluid. They can be used as natural diuretics, which can help to avoid the excessive use of diuretic drugs. Diuretic drugs can be habit forming and the body becomes more resistant to their effect after prolonged or high dosage.

Natural diuretic foods and herbs are:
1. Celery—fresh stalks and seeds
2. Parsley—fresh
3. Dandelion—as coffee or fresh dandelion leaves in salads
4. Fruits containing enzymes such as papaya and pineapple. The enzymes help to soften the stiff and hardened subcutaneous tissues, thereby enhancing the return of retained fluids back to the heart and kidneys. This helps to slim down the limbs.
5. The herbs buchu (200 mg) and horsetail (500 mg)

The dominant gland in the lymphatic type of woman is the pituitary gland situated at the base of the brain (see page 5). The pituitary gland produces several major hormones and its main role is to control the thyroid gland, the adrenals and the ovaries. The pituitary gland can be considered the master gland of the body—controlling, balancing and orchestrating the overall hormonal state.

Some doctors working in the field of obesity believe that an excess of dairy products in the diet causes an overstimulated state of the pituitary gland, which increases the tendency to obesity, especially in lymphatic types. It is true that many lymphatic types of women crave dairy products such as milk, cheese, butter, cream, yogurt, ice cream and chocolate. These foods are not easily metabolized in lymphatic types and predispose to weight gain and excessive mucus.

Many lymphatic women are Caucasian in ancestry and have fair skin, light-colored hair and blue or green eyes. If one examines the iris of the eye, it is easy to see the overburdened lymphatic system in the form of a ring of white dots around the periphery of the colored iris—this is known as a lymphatic rosary (see diagram 8). After a period of dietary cleansing and elimination of dairy products, this lymphatic rosary will clear and the iris will appear brighter and clearer,

Diagram 8

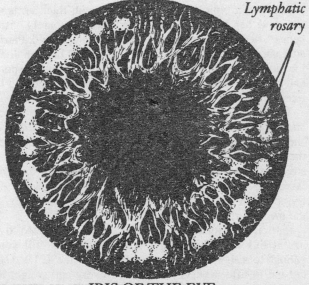

Lymphatic rosary

IRIS OF THE EYE

reflecting its pure blue or green color. The cleansing of the eye's irises reflects the internal cleansing going on in the body after a dairy-free diet such as the Body-Shaping Diet for lymphatic types (see page 121).

PATRICIA'S CASE HISTORY

Patricia had suffered with asthmatic bronchitis for ten years and seemed to be always on antibiotics for another bout of the flu. This made her tired and disinclined to exercise as she felt short of breath and sluggish. She had been slowly gaining weight over the last decade and had put on 33 pounds, which was distributed evenly over her neck, trunk, buttocks, arms and legs. Patricia weighed 159 pounds at a height of 5'3", putting her body mass index at 28.

She was a typical lymphatic shape with thick arms and legs and her wrists and ankle bones were barely visible beneath her subcutaneous tissues swollen with fluid. Patricia complained to me that she felt like a blimpy blob and hated the look and feel of her abdomen and limbs that were spongy and swollen. "Every spring I swell up, gain weight and feel like I am allergic to the twentieth century," she said.

True to lymphatic form, Patricia hated strenuous exercise and loved creamy foods high in dairy products. Little did she know that her high ingestion of dairy foods was one of the main reasons that her immune system could not recover sufficiently to overcome her frequent allergies and viral infections. This was evident by the prominent white dots (lymphatic rosary) around the edge of her blue irises and the swollen rubbery lymph glands in her neck.

Patricia was forty years of age, and I was pleased to see her at this time, knowing that her body was still young enough to respond well to nutritional medicine. If I had seen her ten to fifteen years later, her recovery and weight loss would have been much more difficult and protracted. By this time her immune system may have been damaged so much from her diet, viral infections and repeated courses of antibiotics that it would be impossible to restore to healthy function. Worse still, she may have ended up with autoimmune diseases or severe asthma requiring large doses of cortisone.

Patricia was motivated to change as she not only looked but also felt out of shape. I started her on the Body-Shaping Diet for lymphatic women and asked her to avoid all dairy products and foods with chemical additives. To reduce fluid retention I asked her to eat fresh celery, parsley, dandelion leaves, papaya and pineapple. To improve her resistance to viral infections, I recommended she take vitamin C with bioflavonoids 2000 mg daily along with one or two fresh garlic cloves daily. In those unable to tolerate fresh garlic, odorless garlic capsules are a suitable, although slightly less effective, alternative.

For the first three months on this program, Patricia's body and immune system underwent a cleansing and elimination process. Her daily urinary output increased, her bowel movements became looser and more frequent and she had a greater amount of mucus discharge from her sinuses and lungs. There were days when she felt unwell, complaining on the other end of the phone of headaches and profound fatigue. I reassured her that this was part of her body's catharsis and was to be expected while her body was eliminating deeply buried toxic waste products. During these times I encouraged her to stick to the Body-Shaping Diet, increase her intake of pure water and add half a quart of a mixture of raw carrot, beet, celery and apple juice made daily with a juicer.

By the fourth month she had started to notice big changes—she was no longer wheezing, her bronchial mucus had dried up, her limbs were much slimmer and she had lost 20 pounds. Now that her energy level was increasing I started her on the body-shaping exercise program and reinforced her need to stick to the Body-Shaping Diet and a dairy-free diet.

It took twelve months before Patricia fully recovered and regained her lost shape. She was delighted and said that she had been a thin woman trapped inside a fat woman's body for twenty years. She now weighed 126 pounds with a body mass index between 22 and 23, and the swollen congested layer of fat that had covered her abdomen and limbs was gone. One could now see her bone and muscle structure and her limbs were no longer thick and shapeless.

JOCELYN'S CASE HISTORY

Jocelyn was an inspiring example of how the Body-Shaping Diet and exercise program can change a woman's life. Two years ago, she had been terribly unhappy battling with a weight problem and severe cyclical fluid retention. She was taking strong diuretic and laxative drugs every day to rid herself of swollen legs and feet. These caused mineral imbalances in her body, which resulted in muscle cramps, fatigue and depression.

Jocelyn weighed 172 pounds for a height of 5'1", putting her body mass index at 32. She was disgusted with her thick abdomen, arms and legs, so much so that she wore unattractive baggy clothes to hide herself.

She was a typical lymphatic-shaped woman in that she craved dairy products and salty foods. She had been following a high-protein diet in the mistaken belief that if she avoided sugary sweet foods she must lose weight. Jocelyn had cheese on toast for breakfast, a ham and cheese sandwich for lunch and she loved spaghetti bolognese smothered with salty Parmesan cheese for dinner. She adored olives, salted peanuts, anchovies and salty feta cheese. With such a diet she was retaining so much fluid that she was starting to resemble a bloated jellyfish.

I immediately started Jocelyn on the Body-Shaping Diet for lymphatic women and asked her to avoid all dairy products and salty foods. She was instructed to gradually reduce her dose of diuretic drugs by taking them every second day for one month and then every third day thereafter. I advised that she eat foods high in bioflavonoids, vitamin C and rutosides, such as citrus fruits and buckwheat. I prescribed extracts of the herbs clivers and pokeroot (phytolacca) to strengthen the blood and lymphatic vessels in her limbs.

For the first two weeks Jocelyn actually retained more fluid, especially in her lower legs and gained 4–5 pounds in weight. This was because she had reduced her intake of diuretic drugs resulting in rebound fluid retention. I reassured her that this was only temporary and would pass when her diet and diuretic herbs took effect.

Six weeks after she had started the Body-Shaping Diet, Jocelyn was starting to feel and look much better. The puffiness had gone from her eyes and feet and she now only needed her diuretic tablets twice a week.

I referred her to a physical therapist who gave her the technique of lymphatic massage. The physical therapist massaged her limbs beginning at the fingers and toes and working upward, encouraging excess subcutaneous fluid to move up through the lymphatic vessels. This massage also improved circulation to the fatty layer, thus stimulating the excretion of waste products from the fat. Jocelyn was also doing the exercises in the body-shaping exercise program to stimulate the muscle pump in her limbs.

A physical metamorphosis started to take place in her limbs and after four months I could see her bony and muscular anatomy defining, where previously there had been layers of swollen fatty tissue. After six months, Jocelyn was a new woman both in appearance and demeanor. She weighed 128 pounds and was wearing body-hugging jeans and skirts and was able to wear attractive belts around her now slim and feminine waist. The shy, studious hermit had turned into a social butterfly who was now too busy and full of *joie de vivre* to worry about how she appeared to others.

Two years after our first consultation, Jocelyn met the man of her dreams, at the side of a swimming pool of all places! By this time she looked taut and terrific in a bikini and felt totally relaxed about her uncovered body in public. Thanks to the Body-Shaping Diet, she had found a way to feel good about herself, improve her health and meet a beautiful man to boot!

CHAPTER SEVEN

THE THYROID-SHAPED WOMAN

The thyroid type has long fine-boned limbs and a slender neck and can be described as lean and rangy. She has the racehorse or greyhound look.

Her dominant gland is the thyroid gland, which is the soft fleshy gland situated in front of the neck or Adam's apple. The thyroid gland produces thyroid hormone, which stimulates and controls the metabolic rate. The thyroid-shaped woman when in good health has a high metabolic rate and burns up food calories efficiently. Of all the body shapes, the thyroid is the hardest to fatten and generally these types will be able to eat high-calorie and high-fat foods without gaining weight easily.

Thyroid-shaped women are often nervous types and may be described in colloquial terms as high-strung. They often find it hard to relax and many are workaholics or high achievers. They seem to be always on the go, and their high level of mental and physical activity helps to keep them slim.

On the surface, thyroid-shaped women appear to have abundant energy. However, it is rather superficial and they lack the enduring stamina of android-shaped women. To keep themselves going, thyroid types often crave quick energy boosters and stimulant substances. Many consume sweets and chocolates, coffee, hot spicy foods, cigarettes, diet pills and other stimulants to boost their energy levels when they start to flag. This makes them feel energetic for several hours until they flag again when more stimulants are required. Such stimulant substances cause their thyroid and adrenal glands to pump out more thyroid hormones and adrenal hormones such as cortisone and adrenaline. These hormones produce a temporary high and raise blood sugar levels, which enables the thyroid-type woman to continue her frenetic pace.

If these bad habits continue, eventually the thyroid and adrenal glands suffer from a state of depleted exhaustion and weight gain or chronic fatigue occurs. Once the thyroid and adrenal glands become exhausted, the metabolic rate slows down and weight gain occurs. Fat is deposited upon the abdomen and thighs while the lower parts of the limbs remain relatively slim.

Thyroid-shaped women often miss meals, preferring to snack on quick fixes such as chocolate, coffee and cakes. They also have the highest incidence of eating disorders such as anorexia and bulimia. Lady Diana, Princess of Wales, is a classical thyroid-shaped woman with long slender limbs. She has the typical thyroid personality and has displayed a propensity for eating disorders.

If a thyroid-shaped woman is underweight she will produce lower amounts of estrogen compared to the amounts she produces when her weight falls into the normal range (see the table on page 37). She also has relatively less estrogen than the gynecoid-shaped woman, who tends toward estrogen excess. Because the thyroid-shaped woman tends to be low in estrogen or hypoestrogenic, if she becomes underweight she will lose fat first from the estrogen-dependent areas of her body, namely her breasts, buttocks and upper thighs. Thyroid-shaped women who fall into the underweight or very underweight range (see diagram 5, page

38) often have such low levels of estrogen that their menstrual periods become very infrequent or stop completely. This is most undesirable because, if it persists, the chronically low levels of estrogen increase the risk of osteoporosis and cardiovascular disease. This is because our bones, heart and blood vessels require adequate amounts of estrogen to stay healthy.

I always encourage thyroid-shaped women to take care of their thyroid and adrenal glands by avoiding quick-fix stimulants such as sugar, alcohol or cigarettes. These things will make their blood sugar levels unstable, causing highs and lows in blood sugar—the so-called sugar slippery dip effect. To avoid low blood-sugar levels, they need regular meals containing first-class protein such as fish, meat, dairy products or a combination of grains, nuts, seeds and legumes. The Body-Shaping Diet for thyroid women (see page 129) is designed to provide steady amounts of protein and complex carbohydrates to stabilize blood sugar levels and strengthen the thyroid and adrenal glands. This will avoid the state of chronic thyroid and adrenal exhaustion and resultant obesity that many of these women find themselves in.

Thyroid-shaped women with low levels of estrogen are usually very slim to underweight and may desire to increase the size of their breasts and buttocks—in other words, they may want to look more feminine and curvaceous. To do this, it will be necessary to gain weight and increase the levels of estrogen in the body. The latter can be done with the oral contraceptive pill, which is ideal in younger women requiring regular periods and contraception, or with hormone replacement therapy in older menopausal women. If these methods are not suitable, another strategy to increase body estrogen levels is to consume foods that have a significant content of natural plant estrogen. Estrogenic substances have been discovered in over three hundred different plants and although they are relatively weak, if they are consumed

FOODS CONTAINING NATURAL ESTROGENS

linseed	garlic	green beans	red beans
pumpkin	split peas	marrow	cow peas
olives	olive oil	soybeans	bakers' yeast
parsley	chickpeas	rhubarb	cherry
corn	oats	barley	rye
wheat	rice	peas	sesame
licorice	french beans	clover	red clover
apples	fennel	alfalfa	aniseed
hops	sage	corn oil	sunflower
carrots	beets	plum	squash
cabbage	soy sprouts	potato	yams
			papaya

regularly they may be helpful in boosting the body's estrogen supply.

These foods are high in not only estrogens, but also vitamins, minerals, fatty acids and fiber and are low in saturated fat. Thus there are many good reasons to consume them on a regular basis.

NUTRITIONAL SUPPLEMENTS

There are specific nutritional supplements that act to reduce the tendency to unstable blood sugar levels and reduce the craving for quick sugar fixes that many women suffer with. Over the years I have encountered thousands of sugarholic and chocoholic women who have been helped with nutritional medicine. Indeed, many of them could not believe how their insatiable cravings for sugar were eliminated, so that they rarely thought of bingeing on sugar, while previously they had been tormented by their need for a quick sugar fix. This sugar addiction is most common in the thyroid-shaped woman, but it also occurs to a lesser degree in all the other body shapes.

NUTRITIONAL SUPPLEMENTS REQUIRED TO BEAT THE SUGAR FIX

Vitamins and Minerals

Calcium ascorbate (vitamin C) 1000 mg, niacinamide (vitamin B3) 500 mg, calcium D-pantothenate (vitamin B5) 500 mg, pyridoxine (vitamin B6) 50 mg, thiamine (vitamin B1) 100 mg, riboflavin (vitamin B2) 100 mg, d-alpha tocopherol (vitamin E) 100 I.U., retinol (vitamin A) 5000 I.U., folic acid 400 mcg, cyanocobalamin (vitamin B12) 25 mcg, D-biotin (vitamin H) 25 mcg, potassium citrate 50 mg, magnesium orotate 100 mg, zinc amino acid chelate 20 mg, manganese amino acid chelate 5 mg, chromium amino acid chelate 1 mg.

Amino Acid Tablets Containing

L-glycine, L-proline, L-hydroxyproline, L-glutamic acid, L-alanine, L-arginine, L-aspartic acid, L-serine, L-lysine, L-leucine, L-phenylalanine, L-valine, L-threonine, L-isoleucine, L-hydroxylysine, L-histidine, L-methionine, L-tyrosine. (Take 1 tablet with every meal.)

Thyroid-shaped women suffering with chronic fatigue or obesity will benefit from additional supplements designed to strengthen their thyroid and adrenal glands. These will help the thyroid and adrenal glands to produce steady levels of hormones in the correct balance. The adrenal glands normally produce their peak levels of hormones in the morning, at the start of the day, which is necessary to prepare you for a productive, action-packed day. So if you are feeling particularly poor in the mornings, needing strong coffee or a sugar fix, it is a warning that your adrenal glands are not performing well.

SUPPLEMENTS TO HELP THYROID-SHAPED WOMEN WITH OBESITY AND/OR CHRONIC EXHAUSTION

1. Antioxidant vitamins, e.g., vitamin C 2000 mg daily, beta-carotene 10 mg daily, vitamin E 1000 I.U. daily
2. Evening primrose oil 3000 mg daily
3. Vitamin B5 500 mg and choline 500 mg daily

These nutritional supplements combined with the Body-Shaping Diet and exercise program will benefit thyroid and adrenal gland function. This will regulate the metabolic rate and start the process of weight normalization—either weight gain or weight loss depending on whether you are an underweight or an overweight thyroid shape.

These nutritional supplements should be continued in this dosage for three months. Thereafter you may take them every third day as a maintenance program. Once you are feeling entirely well and feel confident with the Body-Shaping Diet for thyroid women, you may discontinue the supplements. If, however, you wish to continue them, it is quite safe to do so on a maintenance dose (i.e., once every third day).

FUNCTION OF THE THYROID GLAND

When we talk of the function of the thyroid and adrenal glands we are talking in degrees of relative function. We feel really well and metabolize our food efficiently when our glands are functioning at their optimal level. In some women, the function of the thyroid gland gradually and insidiously becomes suboptimal. This causes a slowing of the metabolic rate and a reduction in mental and physical activity with resultant weight gain. A blood test done at this time may still show that thyroid gland function falls in the normal range of the general population, although it is often at the lower limits of this normal range. Such women may be told that their thyroid function is normal and to return in twelve months to repeat the test. Most doctors do not accept that treatment is necessary unless the thyroid function falls below the normal range in a blood test. However, what we need to be aware of is that the present state of function of the thyroid gland is often suboptimal, relative to how it functioned several years ago. Many women, especially thyroid types, are very sensitive to this state of gradual thyroid underactivity and wish to undergo treatment to restore thyroid function before it reaches a level below the normal range in a blood test. In such cases, the nutritional supplements and Body-Shaping Diet for the thyroid woman will help to improve thyroid function.

Once blood tests reveal that the thyroid gland is functioning below the normal range, supplementation with thyroid hormone is necessary. A truly underactive thyroid gland will cause the gradual onset of a collection of unpleasant symptoms. Typically these are a general slowing down of all systems resulting in weight gain around the neck and abdomen associated with a general puffiness of the face, hands and legs and dryness of the skin and hair. The body temperature and pulse rate decrease, the voice deepens and constipation occurs. If thyroid hormone replacement is not given a slowness will develop in speech, nervous reflexes and mental activity.

The usual type of thyroid hormone replacement given is Levoxine, also known as T4, and this is suitable treatment for the majority of women with an underactive thyroid. After commencing Levoxine, the metabolic rate increases and weight loss and a return of well-being should occur.

THYROID RESISTANCE

A small percentage of women with an underactive thyroid find that replacement with Levoxine does not produce weight loss or a state of well-being. This may be due to a state of thyroid resistance when the body does not respond to Levoxine (T4).

Before T4 can be used by the body, it must be converted in our body cells to another form known as T3, which is the more active and potent form of thyroid hormone. In cases of thyroid resistance the body cannot convert T4 to T3 efficiently. This problem can be overcome by giving thyroid hormone replacement in the form of T3 instead of the conventional T4. T3 can be obtained on prescription under the brand name Cytomel.

If you have an underactive thyroid gland and do not feel well or are unable to lose weight by taking Levoxine (T4) tablets, you could ask your doctor about the possibility of changing to or supplementing your Levoxine tablets with Cytomel (T3) tablets. Theoretically, T3 tablets should be more effective in women with a poor response to T4 tablets because they do not need conversion to another form and have a more rapid and powerful effect on the metabolism. Cytomel (T3) tablets are no more expensive than Levoxine (T4) tablets but they need to be given two or three times daily. The starting dose is around 5 micrograms (mcg) twice daily, with a gradual increase to around 20 to 60 mcg daily. Your doctor can adjust the dosage to keep you feeling and looking good and to maintain your blood tests for thyroid function within the normal range. It is important that your dosage of thyroid hormone replacement is carefully controlled; you should always be guided by your own doctor in such cases.

MARIA'S CASE HISTORY

Maria came to see me in a most distressed state. She was a beautiful-looking girl with black hair and an olive complexion and was a typical thyroid shape with long slim limbs. She had come to see me as a last resort, having been to several doctors over the last twelve months seeking help for her underactive thyroid gland.

She had been prescribed thyroid hormone replacement in the form of Levoxine (T4), but it was not helping her symptoms—she remained tired and irritable, her hair and eyebrows were falling out and she could not lose weight.

On examination, she was definitely carrying some excess weight around her abdomen and thighs and weighed 172 pounds at a height of 5'10", giving her a body mass index of approximately 25.

Her doctor had been gradually increasing her dosage of Levoxine (T4) tablets but although her blood tests showed that this dose was resulting in normal thyroid function, her symptoms of hair loss and weight gain remained. She was totally frustrated and depressed.

I suggested that she may have a case of thyroid resistance and that we should try reducing her dose of Levoxine (T4) and supplementing it with some Cytomel (T3). Maria was keen to try anything new and so we embarked on the double-pronged strategy of Levoxine (T4) plus Cytomel (T3). I also asked Maria to change her diet and lifestyle and follow the Body-Shaping Diet and exercise program for the thyroid-shaped woman.

Maria returned after three months and was much happier and energetic than she had been during our first encounter. Her hair and eyebrows had stopped falling out and her chronic fatigue was becoming less each day. She was pleased with the Body-Shaping Diet as she no longer craved sugar and coffee to keep her going.

After six months on this program, Maria felt like her old

self and was pleased to rediscover her slim thyroid shape at a weight of 145 pounds. It was decided in collaboration with her specialist that she would continue both T4 and T3 in a sufficient dose to keep her blood tests for thyroid function in the normal range.

ZOE'S CASE HISTORY

Zoe's husband brought her to see me as he was increasingly concerned about her low body weight, although Zoe herself was not at all perturbed by her rather anorexic-looking body. Zoe was twenty-eight and her weight loss had started after a holiday in Europe, where she had gained 15 pounds, which prompted her friends to comment on her new shape. Although Zoe had never been obese, she was very sensitive to her friends' remarks and she subconsciously decided to lose weight from this point on.

Zoe was a typical thyroid shape, with small bones and long skinny limbs. In true thyroid style, she relied on stimulants such as cigarettes, chocolates and coffee to keep her going during her busy shifts as a nurse in a hospital cardiac unit. She would usually miss breakfast, preferring coffee and a cigarette, and snacked on a chocolate bar at the midmorning break. Lunch consisted of a sandwich. However, Zoe, terrified of gaining weight, would ensure that she ate only one quarter of her sandwich and finished off this paltry meal with coffee and a cigarette.

Zoe's blood sugar levels were understandably quite unstable and around 3:00 P.M. they would plummet, resulting in the need for another chocolate bar. She was a high achiever and very eager to please her colleagues so that she stayed late at work, arriving home around 7:30 P.M. when she would find a tasty healthy meal lovingly prepared by her husband. Despite pleas from her husband, Zoe was lucky to eat half of the food on the plate as during the meal she started to feel guilty and anxious about eating a normal amount of food. The harder her husband tried to encourage her to eat, the more resistant Zoe became until she finally resorted to hiding some of the evening meal so that her husband would believe she had eaten more than she had.

Zoe's history was typical of an underweight thyroid woman. As her weight loss had continued, her estrogen levels had become lower and lower, culminating in the cessation of regular menstrual bleeding. Zoe had not had a period for six months and had lost a lot of weight from the estrogen-sensitive areas of her body—namely, her breasts, buttocks and thighs. She definitely looked anorexic with a weight of 104 pounds at a height of 5'8", giving her a body mass index of 16.

Due to Zoe's self-imposed calorie-restricted diet, which we worked out was around 700 calories per day, her metabolic rate had slowed down as a self-preservation mechanism. This was an automatic reaction of her body to her semistarvation diet. Due to her slow metabolism her hands and feet felt colder than normal, her pulse rate was slow (under 60) and her skin and hair were dry and unhealthy in appearance.

Despite all this, Zoe felt that everything was fine, as she had now developed in her mind a distorted self-image. Although to all outsiders she looked painfully thin, to herself she was a touch overweight and needed to lose all traces of fat.

I was quite worried about Zoe's future in the long term if she continued with her eating patterns, as she would have an increased risk of premature osteoporosis and cardiovascular disease secondary to her low body levels of estrogen.

In all anorexic women there is a high resistance to weight gain and normal eating behavior due to emotional conflicts hidden deep in the subconscious mind. Basically, Zoe suffered from very poor self-esteem and had trouble in asserting her needs. She desperately wanted to enjoy life and be accepted, but was too frightened to really be herself. Her extremely skinny and unfeminine shape protected her from having to fully involve herself with the outside world and men in particular.

I referred Zoe to a psychologist for in-depth counseling and behaviorial therapy so that we could get her to the point where she wanted to accept a normal eating pattern. In Zoe's recovery plan, the emphasis was on eating for well-being, the restoration of normal estrogen levels and supplements that would maintain normal blood sugar levels so that she would no longer need to snack on chocolates and candy. The idea of gaining weight and changing body shape was not emphasized strongly, as these things were far too confronting at this point in her recovery. Zoe needed to feel in control of her body and her destiny and I knew that she would remain underweight for some time, at least until she felt ready to change.

My role was to educate her about her body's needs and how her general health and energy could be helped by regular meals containing protein and complex carbohydrates. In the meantime, I could keep a close eye on her weight and metabolism by seeing her every two weeks. In anorexia nervosa there is a significant risk of severe malnutrition and death and I would need to work hard to acquire and keep her trust and confidence.

As I expected, Zoe's weight fluctuated between 104 pounds and 108 pounds for six months. On her fourteenth visit to me, I could see a change in her mental state and demeanor—she was more relaxed and less exacting of herself and was starting to enjoy eating again. On the fifteenth visit she was menstruating and told me that her breasts had been tender that month—a sure sign that her body estrogen levels were returning to normal. She related that her interest in sex had returned and overall she felt more easygoing and less obsessional about controlling everything in her daily life. In other words she was becoming more trusting about the process of life and was taking time to smell the flowers along the way.

After this time, Zoe's weight gain became automatic and she started steadily gaining around half a pound each week. She would occasionally have a bad week and become tense and anxious about work, which caused her to miss out on breakfast; during these weeks she would lose around one pound in weight.

Zoe's psychologist taught her meditation and techniques of self-visualization where she saw herself easily achieving the goals and desires closest to her heart. These things helped Zoe enormously and eighteen months after our first encounter she had reached a weight of 121 pounds, putting her body mass index at 19. This was just slightly under the desirable weight range for her height and small skeletal frame. I was quite happy with this as Zoe's estrogen levels, menstrual cycle and general metabolism were all back to normal. Zoe was once again enjoying life and now that she had more energy she started the body-shaping exercise program to tone up her arms and legs.

Zoe's case history is typical of many women with anorexia nervosa that I have seen over my years in clinical practice. Anorexia nervosa is a form of self-imposed semistarvation and is more common in thyroid-shaped women. It needs to be handled with great sensitivity, compassion and skill if a cure is to be long lasting.

CLARA'S CASE HISTORY

Clara was a model for a fashion house and was paid handsomely to model a range of swimwear. She had a thyroid-shaped figure with a long fine neck, smallish bone structure and the longest pair of legs I had ever seen.

In typical thyroid style, Clara was addicted to stimulants—she craved caffeine, cigarettes, chocolates and hot spicy Asian foods. She was also addicted to diet pills, which gave her a temporary stimulus and helped her to avoid bingeing on chocolate.

Not surprisingly, Clara suffered extreme mood changes and energy highs and lows, which made it difficult for her to exercise and keep her muscles toned sufficiently to flatter her swimwear range. She was worried by the slow accumulation of fat around her abdomen and upper thighs and came to me seeking help to regain her trim muscular form.

To keep her mood changes under control, Clara's doctor had prescribed antidepressant drugs. However, their sedative effects were not tolerated by Clara's thyroid-type personality, which was accustomed to feeling stimulated and not sedated. These antidepressant drugs also caused her appetite to increase so she had been quick to discard them.

I explained that if we kept her levels of blood sugar, thyroid and adrenal hormones steady, instead of their present wild fluctuations, we could stop her mood swings and fatigue. This would then enable Clara to easily resist her cravings for sugar, coffee and stimulant diet pills.

To achieve these goals Clara was started on the Body-Shaping Diet for thyroid-shaped women and the body-shaping exercise program. This particular diet contains complex carbohydrates and first-class protein in each meal (see menus, page 129) that stabilize blood sugar levels. The Body-Shaping Diet for thyroid women is high in protein, minerals such as calcium, magnesium and iodine and also contains an abundance of estrogenic foods. These ingredients are beneficial for the function of the thyroid gland and help to maintain strong, youthful bones.

Clara was asked to avoid her binges on sugar, coffee, chocolate, cigarettes and very hot spicy meals, as in the long term these stimulants would exhaust her thyroid and adrenal glands, making it very difficult for her to lose weight. To aid her resolution, I prescribed multivitamin and mineral tablets and amino acid tablets, one tablet 3 times daily, as these would stabilize her blood sugar levels and greatly reduce her cravings for stimulant foods and drugs.

To reduce her unpleasant mood changes, which alternated from depression and fits of crying to extreme anger and aggression, I prescribed some single amino acids to be taken with a glass of orange juice at night. These consisted of phenylalanine 800 mg, and glutamine 400 mg. To these I added one vitamin B complex tablet with the evening meal. These nutritional supplements would rebalance the chemicals in her brain cells (neurochemicals) and promote a more stable and efficient mode of mental functioning.

As thyroid types tend to be driven and burn the candle at both ends, I emphasized the need for eight hours of sleep at night, time for relaxation and time to follow the Body-Shaping Diet plan.

Because Clara was only 12 pounds overweight, that is as far as keeping her modeling job was concerned, it only took her five weeks on the Body-Shaping Diet to lose the excess pounds from her abdomen and thighs. She was very grateful for the nutritional supplements because they had stopped her horrible moods and angry outbursts, which were ruining her relationships. They had also enabled her to give up diet pills, Coca-Cola and chocolate, and she thought it fabulous that one could follow a tasty diet, not feel tired and deprived and still lose weight! I replied, "Simply elementary, my dear. Rebalance the hormones and body biochemistry and the weight takes care of itself!"

MIGRAINES

One other point I would like to mention is that migraine headaches occur more frequently in thyroid-shaped women, especially those with the typical thyroid high-achieving or driven personalities. In thyroid-type women who suffer migraines, it is prudent to avoid foods containing the amine called tyramine. Such foods are wine (especially red), beer, chocolate, lima and Italian beans, mature or hard yellow cheeses and indeed all cheeses (except for cottage cheese), chicken liver, raisins, plums, beef liver, chicken skin, herring, sausage, soy sauce, very ripe bananas, pineapple, eggplant, tomato, walnuts, and pecans. This is because tyramine can cause the blood vessels in the brain to constrict and then swell, resulting in migraine headaches.

PART TWO

BODY-SHAPING EATING PLANS

CHAPTER EIGHT

STEP ONE: WEIGHT LOSS

The Body-Shaping Diet is simple and easy to follow and uses a two-step strategy.

Step One of the diet allows you to have 1000 calories each day to achieve maximum weight loss. You will enjoy nutritious and economical meals that require minimal preparation.

Stay within the guidelines for your body type, selecting only those foods recommended and completely avoiding the undesirable foods.

In Step One is a range of sample menus for breakfast, lunch and dinner, suited to each body type, from which you may freely select meals. They are calculated at 1000 calories per day.

Because the basic strategy includes a high intake of carbohydrate foods such as whole grains and starchy vegetables, you will find the meals very satisfying. You will not experience fluctuations in blood sugar levels, which can leave you tired, moody and excessively hungry.

Each body type will have its individual danger periods when you will be tempted to snack. This is explained in detail in later chapters. Have some raw celery, carrots or apples on hand for these occasions.

No other foods should be eaten at these times or weight loss will be slowed down.

While on Step One of the program it is most beneficial for you to follow the exercise program. This will speed weight loss by burning fat and toning muscle tissue. Positive results will show very quickly and you will look and feel lighter, with an increase in energy and vitality.

You may wish to keep a food diary, where you write down all foods eaten each day.

> **Weigh and measure yourself once a week at the same time of day and keep a record. Take measurements of your bust, waist, hips, buttocks, thighs and upper arms. Some weeks, as your body shape and metabolism are changing, you may not lose pounds but you will lose inches.**

When you have reached your desired body weight, move straight on to Step Two—the Maintenance Program designed specifically for your body shape.

STEP TWO: WEIGHT MAINTENANCE

Our maintenance strategy allows you to increase your caloric intake to suit your individual requirements. We have included a range of sample menus for breakfast, lunch and dinner calculated at approximately 1400 calories per day.

Some women will find this too high and may need to keep their caloric intake at 1200 calories per day to maintain a desirable weight. Others who exercise consistently may need a little more than 1400 calories each day.

While following our maintenance strategy you will enjoy the freedom of introducing some healthy desserts (see pages 225) into your diet. You will also increase your fruit and carbohydrate intake.

Staying within the guidelines for your body shape (beginning on page 106) makes it easy for you to maintain your desirable weight and to continue to look and feel healthy and vital.

GENERAL GUIDELINES FOR ALL BODY SHAPES DURING STEPS ONE AND TWO

- **Drink 6 to 8 glasses of water daily.** This includes seltzer, mineral water and herbal teas.
- **Chew your food well.** This is important for the digestion of all foods, particularly fruit, raw vegetables and grains. The nutrients in these foods are surrounded by undigestible cellulose membranes that need to be broken in order for you to utilize the nutrients locked inside. Chewing also triggers the secretion of enzymes that are necessary for the breakdown and utilization of your food. Food that has been chewed well will not irritate the lining of the stomach or the intestines and is digested with ease.
- **Do not drink with meals.** It is important not to interfere with digestion by washing down undigested food with drinks. Try to have your fluids about half an hour before or after meals.
- **Eat in a relaxed environment.** If you are stressed while eating, you are more likely to rush your food, which will lead to difficult digestion and possibly discomfort.
- **Try to eat early in the evening.** Going to bed with a full stomach is often a major contributor to poor sleep patterns. There may also be a large time gap between lunch and dinner and this can lead to binge eating if your blood sugar level is allowed to drop too low.

- **Never skip breakfast.** There are no excuses for avoiding breakfast as it requires minimal preparation. You must provide nutrients, fiber and energy to your body in the morning in order to remain physically and mentally alert, and to avoid mood swings.
- **Shop wisely.** Make sure your refrigerator and pantry are well stocked with healthy food choices. The most economical way to shop is to buy fresh food. The packaged and processed foods are the ones that are often unhealthy, unnecessary and expensive.
- **Maintain a positive attitude.** Set yourself realistic goals that you are able to achieve and try not to dwell on past failures. Live in the present moment.
- **Stay close to nature.** Select foods that do not contain chemical additives, colors or preservatives.

BREAKFAST

The first meal of the day is designed to increase your metabolic rate and to *break* the twelve-hour *fast* that has occurred overnight.

You should be rested and ready to eat a light but substantial meal that contains all the nutrients and energy to sustain the morning's activities.

Remember, while on Step One of the Body-Shaping Diet, even at breakfast you must take care to eat the correct balance of foods for your body shape.

If you prefer to design your own menu, simply check the amount of calories recommended for your body type, follow your guidelines and create a breakfast that includes a carbohydrate food like cereal or toast, some protein such as low-fat dairy products, eggs, fish, soy milk, etc., a serving of fruit (see page 256) and a beverage of your choice.

Eating breakfast will reduce the temptation to snack midmorning.

LUNCH

Lunch can vary greatly according to your daily routine. Whether it simply consists of a salad, sandwich or a more elaborate business lunch, **by making the right choices it will always be possible to follow your guidelines and achieve weight loss**.

Try not to eat a late lunch or you will experience a drop in blood sugar. If this happens it can turn someone with tremendous willpower into a creature who will devour anything to obtain a quick sugar fix.

If designing your own lunch menu, check your caloric allowance for lunch and the guidelines for your body shape.

Have a small serving of protein (page 249) and adequate carbohydrate (page 238). Always include lots of green leafy vegetables or salad to assist with digestion and to add nutrients. You may eat your fruit serving with lunch or save it for an afternoon snack.

MAIN MEAL OF THE DAY

Whether you have your main meal at lunch or in the evening it must include a serving of a complete protein food, carbohydrate food and green vegetable or salad.

PROTEIN

Meat 3.5 ounces. Must be lean with all visible fat removed before cooking. Approximately **180 calories**. DO NOT FRY.

Chicken 3.5 ounces. Remove all visible fat and skin before cooking. DO NOT FRY. Serving size is approximately ½ chicken breast, which is about **125 calories**.

Fish 3.5 ounces. Approximately **100 calories**. DO NOT FRY.

Soybeans (cooked). 1 cup is approximately **200 calories**.

The only legumes that are complete protein foods are soybeans. Incomplete proteins are chickpeas, navy beans, light red kidney beans, red kidney beans, lentils, brown rice, millet and barley. These should be combined to form a complete protein meal, such as mixing chickpeas and tahini (sesame paste) to make hummus, which is a complete protein. Or make a complete protein meal with Dahl (page 210) and rice and vegetables.

Your recommended serving size for cooked legumes is 1 cup.

At your main meal, as well as your protein, have **two or three servings of starchy vegetables**. Choices are as follows:

1 SERVING

= **1 small baked potato (3 ounces)**	**(90 calories)**
= **¼ cup sweet potato**	**(86 calories)**
= **½ cup mashed potatoes**	**(111 calories)**
= **½ cup beets**	**(22 calories)**
= **½ cup carrots**	**(35 calories)**
= **½ cup cauliflower**	**(20 calories)**
= **¼ cup peas**	**(30 calories)**
= **1 small corn on the cob**	
(2 ounces)	**(62 calories)**
= **½ large parsnip**	**(50 calories)**

If you are having pasta or rice with your meal, it replaces your servings of starchy vegetable. This means that you are allowed to eat the pasta or rice with some protein and unlimited green vegetable or salad.

CARBOHYDRATE

1 SERVING = 2 to 3 STARCHY VEGETABLES
OR
= 1 CUP COOKED PASTA (approximately 160 calories)
OR
= ¾ CUP COOKED RICE (approximately 160 calories)

> **ALWAYS SERVE WITH UNLIMITED GREEN VEGETABLE OR SALAD.** These greens provide necessary nutrients and fiber and need to be eaten every day. Always have at least two servings of green vegetable. They are very low in calories and will speed your weight loss.

Try not to have bread with the main meal of the day. Your fruit serving may be eaten at any time.

THE WEIGHT LOSS PLATEAU

While following the Body-Shaping Diet, there will be times when your weight will stabilize. According to the scales it may not change for a number of weeks.

Maintain your enthusiasm and know that this is a period of transition.

Keep in mind that your body is undergoing a process of change. It takes time to break down stubborn areas where fat cells have been deposited. At the same time your increased exercise helps to build muscle tissue, which is heavier than fat.

While your body changes shape, weight loss may stand still periodically. In women who have been very overweight for many years, the weight-loss plateau may last several months, but weight loss will surely recommence if you continue the Body-Shaping Diet. In such cases it may take one to two years to lose all your excess fat; however, be patient, as the long-term outcome is better this way.

However, reassure yourself it is quite natural to reach a plateau phase when following a weight-loss program. Exercise, sensible eating and a positive attitude will produce the desired result and weight loss will return after the plateau phase, unless you have already reached your body's ideal weight.

CHAPTER NINE

ANDROID SHAPE
EATING PLAN

If you fall into this category you will find that many weight-loss diets don't work for you, especially if they encourage a high intake of protein and a reduction of bread, cereals and starchy vegetables.

Your diet needs to be high in raw fruits, fresh vegetables and whole grains. Protein should come from pulses, legumes, nuts, seeds, fish and low-fat dairy products. You may also include some free-range chickens and eggs in your weekly regime and occasionally some lean red meats.

A semivegetarian diet sits well with you and I have included some vegetarian meals in your sample menus. You will find the vegetarian recipes very easy to prepare and they will supply you with adequate first-class protein.

If you become very overweight, you may face some serious health risks such as diabetes, cardiovascular disease, high blood pressure and high blood cholesterol. I have considered these while planning your eating program.

You will start the day with a light, nutritious breakfast containing fruit, cereal or whole grain toast and low-fat dairy products or low-fat soy milk.

Lunch is also kept light with an emphasis on soups, salads, bread, grains, seeds, nuts, pasta, legumes and fruit. This will keep your appetite under control and rebalance the glands in your body. You cannot alter your adrenal dominance by simply reducing animal products and salt. You must also eat foods to stimulate the liver and so improve your ability to metabolize cholesterol and break down excessive steroid hormones.

Cereals, grains and low-fat dairy products stimulate the thyroid and pituitary glands. This will improve your metabolic rate, regulate hormonal imbalance and open up your creative thought processes.

Late afternoon is often the time when you experience fatigue and hunger. Cheese, crackers and salted peanuts are not the answer, even though the craving for these foods will be strong. You must also avoid the temptation to have an alcoholic drink. This will add unnecessary and useless calories and place added stress on your liver.

For a late afternoon snack have some raw vegetables, such as celery and carrots with an avocado dip, or a small bowl of vegetable soup, or a handful of raw almonds. You will not have to wait long for your dinner, which will be substantial and very satisfying.

STEP ONE:
WEIGHT LOSS FOR THE
ANDROID BODY SHAPE

On waking have a large glass of water with a squeeze of lemon or lime juice.

ANDROID GUIDELINES

FOOD GROUPS	DESIRABLE FOODS	UNDESIRABLE FOODS
Grains, cereal, bread and pasta	Whole grains such as brown rice, millet, barley, wheat, rye, rolled oats, corn, buckwheat. Bread, crispbread, crackers, flour and pasta containing these whole grains.	Highly refined and bleached white flour products such as white bread, packaged cakes and cookies. Avoid products made from white cake flour or bread flour.
Legumes	All beans, lentils and peas. Tofu. All bean sprouts.	
Meat, chicken, game and fish	Fresh and canned fish. Free-range chickens, turkeys and eggs. Occasional lean red meats.	Shellfish and oysters. Commercially raised hens and eggs. Organ meat. Anchovies, processed luncheon meats, bacon, sausages, fried meats.
Dairy products	Low-fat milk, cheese and yogurt. Sheep and goats' milk and yogurt. Rice Dream milk and soy milk.	All full-fat dairy products, including chocolate, cream, cheese, butter and ice cream. Coconut milk.

ANDROID GUIDELINES (cont'd.)

FOOD GROUPS	DESIRABLE FOODS	UNDESIRABLE FOODS
Fruit and vegetables	All fresh or dried fruits, canned fruit in natural juice or water. A wide variety of fresh vegetables.	Fruit in sugar syrup, glazed fruit. Olives.
Nuts and seeds	Unsalted raw nuts and seeds. Tahini and raw nut pastes.	Peanuts and salted nuts. Coconut. Peanut butter.
Fats and oils	Small amounts of olive, linseed and canola oil.	Meat drippings, butter, lard, margarine.
Beverages	Water: 6 to 12 glasses. Mineral water and seltzer. Some herb teas (tannin-free). 1 to 2 cups coffee per day.	Carbonated soft drinks. Cocktails. Malted milk drinks. Alcohol. Tea (green, black or oolong). Chocolate drinks.
Miscellaneous	Very small amounts of honey, sugar or molasses.	Refined sugars and products containing sugars. MSG. Salt and salty foods. Artificial additives, preservatives and colors.

BREAKFAST

Select any **one** of the following choices.
EACH SELECTION = APPROXIMATELY
250 CALORIES

- ¾ cup fresh berries, 1 cup low-fat 2% plain yogurt, 2 teaspoons LSA (see page 263). Cup of herbal tea.
- 1 ounce breakfast cereal (page 242), 4 ounces low-fat calcium-enriched milk, ½ tablespoon each lecithin and LSA (page 263). 6 medium strawberries.
- 2 slices dry whole grain toast with ¼ cup low-fat 2% cottage cheese, sliced tomato and alfalfa sprouts. 1 nectarine.
- ¾ cup cooked rolled oats with 4 ounces low-fat 2% calcium-enriched milk, soy milk or Rice Dream milk and ½ cup sliced strawberries and banana, ½ tablespoon each LSA (page 263) and wheat germ.
- 2 slices dry whole grain toast with 2 ounces fresh roasted turkey. 1 kiwifruit.
- Your choice of a small piece of fresh fruit blended with 4 ounces low-fat calcium-enriched 2% milk or Rice Dream milk, ice cubes and 1 teaspoon lecithin and wheat germ. 1 slice raisin bread.
- 1 poached or boiled egg with 1 slice dry whole grain toast. 8 ounces fresh orange juice.
- 1 Apple and Oat Bran Muffin (page 226), 1 large piece fresh fruit of your choice. Cup of herbal tea.
- 1 toasted whole wheat English muffin spread with a ¼ cup low-fat 2% cottage cheese. 1 sliced kiwifruit and 6 strawberries.
- 1 slice dry whole grain toast topped with ¼ avocado, ½ freshly sliced tomato, chopped chives and freshly ground black pepper. 1 cup cantaloupe or honeydew cubes.

LUNCH

Select any **one** of the following choices
**EACH SELECTION = APPROXIMATELY
350 CALORIES**

- ½ cup Guacamole (page 171), served with 3 cups mixed fresh raw vegetables such as radish, fennel, carrot, zucchini, green pepper, celery and broccoli florets. 1 large serving fresh fruit.
- ½ pita bread (1 ounce) with 1 Oven-Baked Falafel (page 196), 1 tablespoon Hummus (page 171), lettuce and ½ cup Tabbouli Salad (page 176). ½ cup berries.
- Whole grain bread roll (2 ounces) with fresh green salad, 1 tomato, ½ cup raw grated beets and ¼ medium avocado. Small bunch of grapes.
- 2 cups Italian Noodle Soup (page 175), green salad including 1 cup mixed raw vegetables with No Oil Dressing (page 189), 2 whole wheat saltine crackers. 1 large serving fresh fruit or juice.
- 3.5 ounces pink salmon and ¼ cup 2% fat cottage cheese with a large garden salad with 3 tablespoons Mustard Vinaigrette (page 188) and ½ cup beets. 1 cup cantaloupe cubes.
- 3 sesame Ryvita with ⅓ cup whole milk ricotta cheese, 3 oil-packed drained, chopped sardines, fresh tomato slices, onion and fresh parsley. 2 slices fresh pineapple (approximately ½ cup).
- 1 serving Pasta Salad (page 179), 1 small baked potato. 8 ounces apple juice.
- 1 cup Minestrone Soup (page 173), garden salad with 1 cup sliced beets, 1 whole grain bread roll (2 ounces). Small bunch of grapes.
- 1 serving Quick Curried Eggs (page 211), garden salad with No Oil Dressing (page 189). 1 large serving fresh fruit or juice.

- 1 serving Fresh Asparagus Vinaigrette (page 177), 1 medium baked potato with 2 tablespoons Mock Sour Cream Dressing (page 190), 2 whole wheat saltine crackers. 1 medium peach.
- 1 serving Low-Calorie Cannelloni (page 213), garden salad with 2 tablespoons Mustard Vinaigrette (page 188), 1 cup beets. 1 small serving fresh fruit or juice.
- 1 cup Squash Soup (page 174), 1 slice rye bread, 1 cup Mushroom and Snow Pea Salad (page 183). 1 cup watermelon balls.

EVENING

Select any **one** of the following choices.
**EACH SELECTION = APPROXIMATELY
400 CALORIES**

- 3.5 ounces grilled white fish with 1 serving Tomato Salsa (page 195), 1 medium baked potato with 2 teaspoons Mock Sour Cream Dressing (page 190), green salad with No Oil Dressing (page 189). ½ cup fruit salad.
- 1 serving Fruit and Chicken Salad (page 186), ½ cup cooked brown rice, 2 cups Cucumber Salad (page 186).
- Green Vegetable Plate (2 cups) with 1 tablespoon Dukkah (page 178), 1 cup Dahl (page 210), ½ cup cooked brown rice. ½ sliced banana with ½ cup raspberries.
- 2 small taco shells filled with 2 servings Quick Mexican Beans (page 209), fresh chopped tomato, shredded lettuce, alfalfa sprouts, 2 tablespoons plain low-fat yogurt and Chili Sauce (page 192). 1 large piece fresh fruit of your choice.
- Lentil Patty (page 208) on a whole grain bread roll (2 ounces) with salad and sprouts, 2 tablespoons Hazelnut

Dressing (page 190), Chili Sauce (page 192). 2 slices fresh pineapple (approximately ½ cup).

- 1 serving Braised Steak (page 200), ¼ cup cooked brown rice. Small serving fresh fruit of your choice.
- 1 serving Alternative Cannelloni (page 214), ¼ cup sweet potato, ½ cup carrots, ½ cup cauliflower, ¼ cup green peas, ½ cup lightly cooked mushrooms. 1 small piece of fresh fruit.
- Baked Stuffed Fish (page 198), 1 small baked potato with 2 tablespoons Mock Sour Cream Dressing (page 190), garden salad with No Oil Dressing (page 189).
- 1 cup cooked spaghetti with 1 serving Pesto Sauce (page 193), garden salad with No Oil Dressing (page 189). 1 large serving fresh fruit.
- 1 serving Chicken and Mushroom Pie (page 203), ½ cup carrots. 1 small serving fresh fruit.
- 3.5 ounces grilled veal loin with 1 serving Napolitana Sauce (page 216), 1 small baked potato, garden salad with No Oil Dressing (page 189). 1 small serving fresh fruit.
- 2 Cabbage Rolls (page 205), ¼ cup sweet potato, ½ cup carrots, ¼ cup peas, ¼ cup green beans. 1 small serving fresh fruit.

GYNECOID SHAPE EATING PLAN

From clinical experience I have observed that gynecoid-shaped women usually skip breakfast or simply enjoy a tea and toast–type breakfast. They will often comment that once they start to eat a heavy meal in the mornings, they find it hard to stop and will binge all day. Whereas if they eat lightly in the morning and have a small lunch they usually feel much lighter and are able to keep their weight under control.

They seem to save up all day and let loose in the evening when some women eat in excess of 1000 calories just having dinner––with wine, followed by dessert, then coffee or tea with a couple of cookies, then . . . for some, the evenings are a total disaster.

Is it any wonder that they often sleep badly and wake up tired? They feel bloated and heavy and are usually prone to constipation due to an overindulgence of food in the evenings and no fiber for breakfast to help push through last night's meal.

I encourage you to keep breakfast and lunch light, as long as they are nutritious and provide your body with the necessary fiber. You will see from the sample menus provided that this is encouraged.

You must never skip breakfast because your first danger period for snacking is late morning. Without breakfast your blood sugar levels will be low and you will be ready for a quick fix at morning break time. This is when you are more likely to go for cookies or cake with coffee or tea. Instead, you should be having a glass of water, natural mineral water or herb tea with a piece of fruit if you are hungry.

Our lunchtime menus are satisfying and nutritious. They are flexible and easy, whether at home, at work or eating out.

Try to have dinner early in the evening so the gap from lunch to dinner is not too long.

If you must eat late, save a fruit serving for early evening or chew some raw salad vegetables until dinner is ready. They are low in calories and easily digested.

> Your evening meal is the largest of the day because this is when your metabolism is most active. You enjoy eating in the evenings and so I have designed an eating plan that presents you with a generous and tasty meal that will not leave you hungry.

Your second danger period is late at night when you tend to look for comfort foods. However, our evening meals are especially designed to satisfy you so that your cravings at this time are minimal. If you must eat something, simply stick to raw fruits and vegetables.

GYNECOID GUIDELINES

FOOD GROUPS	DESIRABLE FOODS	UNDESIRABLE FOODS
Grains, cereal, bread and pasta	Whole grains such as brown rice, corn, rye, wheat, buckwheat, oats, millet and barley. Bread and pasta containing these whole grains.	Highly refined and bleached white flour products such as white bread, packaged cakes and crackers and cookies. Avoid products made from white cake flour or bread flour.
Legumes	Most beans, lentils and peas.	Soybeans, tofu, and bean sprouts are high in plant estrogens, so eat in moderation.
Meat, chicken, game and fish	Choose lean cuts of red meats and trim off fat before cooking. Free-range chickens, turkeys and eggs. Fresh and canned fish.	Processed luncheon meats, bacon, sausages, fried foods. Skin on poultry. Commercially raised hens and eggs. Organ meats.
Dairy products	Low-fat milk, cheese and yogurt. Rice Dream milk.	Full-fat dairy products including butter, cream, ice cream, cheese and chocolate. Coconut milk.

GYNECOID GUIDELINES (cont'd.)

FOOD GROUPS	DESIRABLE FOODS	UNDESIRABLE FOODS
Fruit and vegetables	All fresh and dried fruits, canned fruit in natural juice or water. A wide variety of fresh vegetables.	Fruit in sugar syrup, glazed fruit.
Nuts and seeds	Unsalted raw nuts and seeds. Tahini and raw nut pastes.	Peanuts and salted nuts. Peanut butter. Coconut.
Fats and oils	Small amounts of olive, linseed and canola oil. Dairy-free margarine in moderation only.	Meat drippings, butter, butter blends and lard. Peanut, sunflower, corn, safflower and corn oils.
Beverages	Water: 6 to 12 glasses. Mineral water and seltzer. Cereal beverages (Postum, Ovaltine). Herb teas. 1 to 2 cups coffee per day.	Carbonated soft drinks. Alcohol. Green, black, oolong tea. Chocolate drinks.
Miscellaneous	Very small amounts of honey, sugar or molasses.	Refined sugars and products containing sugar. MSG. Salt and salty foods. Artificial additives, preservatives and colors.

STEP ONE:
WEIGHT LOSS FOR THE
GYNECOID BODY SHAPE

On waking have a large glass of water with a squeeze of lemon or lime juice.

BREAKFAST

Select any **one** of the following choices.
**EACH SELECTION = APPROXIMATELY
250 CALORIES**

- ⅔ cup cooked brown rice, 4 ounces low-fat 2% calcium-enriched milk or soy milk, 2 teaspoons wheat germ. 6 small or 3 large strawberries.
- ¾ cup cooked rolled oats, 4 ounces low-fat 2% calcium-enriched milk, skim milk or low-fat soy milk, sprinkled with 1 tablespoon roasted sesame and sunflower seeds. ½ large or 1 small banana.
- 1 poached or boiled egg, 1 slice dry whole grain toast topped with fresh chopped parsley, 2 slices fresh tomato, snow pea sprouts. 8 ounces fresh orange juice.
- Fruit shake—your choice of a small serving of fresh fruit, blended with 6 ounces skim milk, low-fat 2% calcium-enriched milk, low-fat soy milk or Rice Dream milk, ice cubes and ½ tablespoon each LSA (page 263) and wheat germ. 1 slice of raisin bread.
- 2 slices dry whole grain toast topped with ¼ avocado, sprinkled with lemon juice and ground black pepper.
- 1 ounce breakfast cereal (page 242), 4 ounces skim milk, low-fat 2% calcium-enriched milk or low-fat soy milk or Rice Dream milk, 2 teaspoons wheat germ. 1 small piece of fresh fruit.

- 2 Whole Wheat Pancakes (page 225), ½ small sliced banana, ½ cup raspberries.
- 1 Banana and Pecan Muffin (page 227). 1 serving of fresh fruit of your choice. Cup of herbal tea.
- 1 dry toasted whole wheat English muffin topped with 1 medium fresh tomato, parsley and freshly ground black pepper. ½ cup unsweetened canned peaches.
- 1 slice dry whole grain toast with ½ cup low-fat 2% cottage cheese. ½ cup cantaloupe cubes.

LUNCH

Select any **one** of the following choices.
**EACH SELECTION = APPROXIMATELY
300 CALORIES**

- 2 rice cakes with 3.5 ounces red salmon, sliced tomato, ½ cup sliced beets and unlimited green salad. ½ cup cantaloupe cubes.
- ¼ avocado and lettuce sandwich on 2 slices whole grain bread spread with 1 teaspoon tahini. 1 mandarin orange.
- Whole grain roll (2 ounces) with 1 sliced hard-boiled egg, lettuce, sprouts, 4 thin slices cucumber and 1 teaspoon reduced-fat mayonnaise. 1 small serving of fruit or juice.
- 1 cup Zucchini Soup (page 174) with a whole grain roll (2 ounces) and small green salad with No Oil Dressing (page 189). 1 nectarine.
- Omelet made from 2 medium eggs with 1 tablespoon low-fat milk or soy milk, 5 halved cherry tomatoes, ½ cup chopped fresh mushrooms, chopped chives or shallots, 2 teaspoons chopped parsley, sprinkle of paprika if desired. 3 whole wheat saltine crackers. Small bunch of grapes.
- 2 ounces sardines in spring water, drained, 1 tablespoon

cream cheese, sliced tomato and unlimited green salad with No Oil Dressing (page 189). 2 Ryvita crackers. 1 small serving of fruit or juice.

- ½ pita bread (1 ounce) with 1 tablespoon of Hummus (page 164) or ¼ cup of low-fat 2% cottage cheese, salad of your choice with No Oil Dressing (page 189), 1 Oven-Baked Falafel (page 207). 1 large serving of fruit or juice.
- ½ grilled chicken breast with large garden salad and ¼ cup Mustard Vinaigrette (page 188), 1 cup grated sliced beets mixed with lemon juice. 2 slices fresh pineapple (approximately ½ cup).
- 6 Stuffed Mushroom Caps (page 169), 1 small baked potato with 2 teaspoons Mock Sour Cream Dressing (page 190), garden salad with No Oil Dressing (page 189). 1 cup cantaloupe cubes.
- 1 small baked potato with 1 serving Pesto Sauce (page 193), 1 cup beets, garden salad with No Oil Dressing (page 189). 1 large serving of fruit or juice.
- 1 cup cooked pasta spirals with ½ cup chopped fresh mushrooms, 3 halved cherry tomatoes, ¼ cup chopped green pepper, ½ cup snow peas, parsley and 1 teaspoon chopped pine nuts. Add 1 tablespoon Vinaigrette Dressing (page 189) and mix well. 1 kiwifruit.
- 3.5 ounces grilled whitefish, garden salad with No Oil Dressing (page 189), 1 small baked potato topped with ½ tablespoon Mock Sour Cream Dressing (page 190). ½ cup unsweetened fruit cocktail.

EVENING

Select any **one** of the following choices.
EACH SELECTION = APPROXIMATELY 450 CALORIES

- 3.5 ounces lean, grilled flank steak, 1 serving Chili Sauce (page 192), 1 small sweet potato, 1 cup steamed cauliflower. 1 small serving of fresh fruit.

- ½ grilled chicken breast topped with fresh lime juice, chopped fresh ginger and tarragon, if desired. 1 small baked potato with 2 teaspoons Mock Sour Cream Dressing (page 190). 1 cup sliced beets, a large green salad, including 1 medium grated carrot and 1 sliced fresh tomato. 1 cup unsweetened canned peaches.
- 1 serving Irish Stew (page 201), green salad with No Oil Dressing (page 189). 1 small bunch grapes (approximately 30).
- 1 Creamy Fish Roll with Dill Sauce (page 197), 1 medium baked potato, 1 cup carrots, 8 brussels sprouts. 1 medium orange.
- 1 serving Low-Calorie Cannelloni (page 213), 1 small corn on the cob, 1 small sweet potato, ½ cup carrots, unlimited green salad with No Oil Dressing (page 189). 1 cup sliced banana and strawberries.
- 2 cups Minestrone Soup (page 173), 1 whole grain roll (2 ounces), 1 small baked potato, 1 cup sliced beets and unlimited garden salad with No Oil Dressing (page 189). ½ cup cantaloupe cubes.
- 1 serving Butternut and Cashew Quiche (page 210), ½ cup steamed cauliflower with ¼ cup Parsley Sauce (page 193), ½ cup steamed carrots, garden salad with No Oil Dressing (page 189). 1 cup watermelon balls.
- 2 Cabbage Rolls (page 205), 1 small baked potato, ¾ cup squash, 12 snow peas. 1 small serving of fresh fruit.
- 1 serving Lamb and Fruit Kebabs (page 199), Spinach and Walnut Salad (page 181).
- 1 cup cooked spaghetti with 1 serving Pesto Sauce (page 193), garden salad with 4 carrot sticks and 1 tablespoon Vinaigrette Dressing (page 189). 1 medium pear.
- 1 serving Baked Stuffed Fish (page 198), ½ cup mashed potato, ½ cup green beans, 1 medium sliced tomato. ½ cup berries.

- 1 serving Marinated Scallops (page 184) with ⅔ cup cooked brown rice, 1 cup Cucumber Salad (page 186). 2 slices pineapple (approximately ½ cup).

LYMPHATIC SHAPE EATING PLAN

Your body type is prone to weight excess but with perseverance you will achieve the most rewarding results. Because of lymphatic congestion you may tire easily, are prone to increased mucus production and swollen glands. If you continue to follow a diet that contains dairy products, salt and processed foods, your obesity will gradually increase over the years.

I have designed an eating plan for you that will stimulate your sluggish metabolism and circulation and improve your liver and kidney function, resulting in more efficient elimination. It will also liberate your congested lymphatic system.

The best time for you to eat is in the mornings and at lunchtime when your metabolism is most active.

You will enjoy an ample breakfast as this is the best time for your body type and you will remain alert and energetic throughout the morning.

Lunch is to be your main meal of the day. Your metabolism will cope well with food at this time. Within the sample menus you will find a good

selection of protein and carbohydrate foods to keep your blood sugar levels stable throughout the afternoon.

You must always include a raw or steamed green vegetable and salad with your meals to assist the digestive processes. For instance, never settle for pasta with a sauce alone; always include a green salad with it. If you are having soup with a whole wheat roll, eat some salad vegetables as well.

Your danger period will be late afternoon when you start to feel tired. You may experience false hunger at this time and may be tempted to break your diet. To give in and eat fast food or dairy products (which you will naturally crave) will slow down your progress.

With your body type, even the addition of some cottage cheese is enough to stop changes in body shape and well-being.

Your best snack is raw celery, carrot and apple. I also encourage you to drink fresh vegetable juices. Some good choices are: carrot and celery, carrot and apple, carrot, celery and beet, carrot and watermelon. These are great for your kidneys, liver and the elimination of cellulite.

Eat a small meal in the evening when your metabolism is sluggish. You will enjoy a peaceful night's sleep and wake feeling refreshed and much lighter.

STEP ONE:
WEIGHT LOSS FOR THE
LYMPHATIC BODY SHAPE

On waking have a large glass of water with a squeeze of lemon or lime juice.

LYMPHATIC GUIDELINES

FOOD GROUPS	DESIRABLE FOODS	UNDESIRABLE FOODS
Grains, cereal, bread and pasta	Whole grains such as brown rice, corn, rye, wheat, buckwheat, oats, millet and barley. Bread, crispbread, crackers, flour and pasta containing these whole grains.	Highly refined and bleached white flour products such as white bread, packaged cakes and cookies. Avoid products made from white cake flour or bread flour.
Legumes	All beans, lentils and peas. Bean sprouts. Tofu.	
Meat, chicken, game and fish	Choose lean cuts of red meat and trim off fat before cooking. Free-range chickens, turkeys and eggs. Fresh and canned fish. Shellfish and oysters.	Processed luncheon meats, bacon, sausages, fried foods. Commercially raised hens and eggs. Skin on poultry. Organ meats. Anchovies.
Dairy products	None allowed, so substitute with Rice Dream milk low-fat soy milk and soy products.	All dairy products including cream, cheese, butter, ice cream, milk, yogurt and chocolate. Sheep and goats' milk products. Coconut milk.
Fruit and	All fresh and dried fruits, canned fruit in	Fruit in sugar syrup. Glazed fruit.

LYMPHATIC GUIDELINES (cont'd.)

FOOD GROUPS	DESIRABLE FOODS	UNDESIRABLE FOODS
vegetables	natural juice or water. A wide variety of fresh vegetables.	Olives.
Nuts and seeds	Unsalted raw nuts and seeds. Tahini and raw nut pastes.	Peanuts and salted nuts. Peanut butter. Coconut.
Fats and oils	Small amounts of dairy-free margarine and olive oil. Linseed and canola oil, in moderation only.	Meat drippings, butter, butter blends, suet and lard. Margarine.
Beverages	Water: 6 to 12 glasses. Mineral water and seltzer. Cereal beverages (Postum, Ovaltine). Herb teas. 1 to 2 cups coffee per day.	Carbonated soft drinks. Cocktails. Malted milk drinks. Alcohol. Green, black, oolong tea. Chocolate drinks.
Miscellaneous	Very small amounts of honey, sugar or molasses.	Refined sugars and products containing sugars. MSG. Salt and salty foods. Artificial additives, preservatives and colors.

BREAKFAST

Select any **one** of the following choices.
EACH SELECTION = APPROXIMATELY
300 CALORIES

- 1 ounce breakfast cereal (page 242) with 4 ounces soy milk or Rice Dream milk. Add 2 teaspoons oat bran and 1 tablespoon mixed roasted sesame and sunflower seeds, ½ banana and 3 strawberries.
- 1 cup cooked oats with 4 ounces Rice Dream milk or soy milk. ½ cup fresh berries and 2 teaspoons LSA (page 263).
- ½ cup unsweetened canned peaches blended with 4 ounces soy milk or Rice Dream milk, ice cubes and ½ tablespoon each lecithin, wheat germ and oat bran. 1 slice raisin bread.
- 1 slice dry whole grain toast with ¼ medium avocado topped with fresh lime or lemon juice and black pepper. 8 ounces fresh orange juice, 1 medium peach.
- 1 poached egg on 1 slice dry whole grain toast. Pour over 4 tablespoons Blender Hollandaise (page 192) and fresh parsley. May be served with fresh tomato and sprouts. 1 cup cantaloupe cubes.
- 1 slice dry whole grain toast with 3 ounces fresh turkey breast. 6 ounces apple juice.
- 2 Whole Wheat Pancakes (page 225) with 1 banana and 3 strawberries. Cup of tea.
- 2 Apple and Oat Bran Muffins (page 226). Cup of tea.
- 1 toasted whole wheat English muffin spread thinly with 1 tablespoon diet margarine and 2 teaspoons spreadable fruit. 1 small serving of fruit or juice.
- 2 slices dry toasted rye bread with 2 ounces pink salmon, thinly sliced. Serve with sliced fresh tomato. 1 small serving of fruit or juice.

LUNCH

Select any **one** of the following choices.
**EACH SELECTION = APPROXIMATELY
400 CALORIES**

- 2 Quick Curried Eggs (page 211) with green salad and No Oil Dressing (page 189), 2 slices dry whole grain toast. 1 kiwifruit.
- 3.5 ounces pink salmon, 4 Ryvita crackers, green salad with No Oil Dressing (page 189). 1 large serving of fresh fruit or juice.
- 3.5 ounces fresh baked or grilled whitefish, 1 serving Tomato Salsa (page 195), 1 small potato, 1 serving Mushroom and Snow Pea Salad (page 183). 1 small serving of fresh fruit or juice.
- 3.5 ounces lean grilled flank steak with 1 serving Chili Sauce (page 192), 1 cup peas and carrots. 1 small serving of fresh fruit or juice.
- Lentil Patty (page 208) on whole grain roll (2 ounces) with garden salad with No Oil Dressing (page 189), 1 cup sliced beets and grated medium carrot. 2 slices fresh or unsweetened pineapple (approximately ½ cup).
- 1 cup cooked pasta spirals combined with 2 teaspoons Mustard Vinaigrette (page 188), 3.5 ounces tuna in spring water (drained) and 2 cups chopped celery, mushrooms, broccoli, tomato, shallots and artichoke hearts.
- ½ pita bread (1 ounce) filled with 1 Oven-Baked Falafel (page 207), 1 tablespoon Hummus (page 171), ¼ avocado, green salad with No Oil Dressing (page 189). 1 large serving of fresh fruit or juice.
- ¼ avocado and a mixed salad that includes 1 cup sliced beets and 1 grated medium carrot, a whole grain roll (2 ounces). 1 small serving of fresh fruit or juice.
- ½ grilled chicken breast with 1 serving Chili Sauce (page 192), garden salad with fresh lemon juice, 1 small

corn on the cob and 1 small baked potato. 2 slices fresh pineapple (approximately ½ cup).

- 1 cup of cooked spaghetti with 1 serving Pesto Sauce (page 193) and garden salad with fresh lemon juice. 1 large serving of fresh fruit or juice.
- 1 cup Minestrone Soup (page 173), 1 whole grain muffin (2 ounces), Green Vegetable Plate (approximately 2 cups) with 2 tablespoons Dukkah (page 178). 1 small serving of fresh fruit.
- 1 serving Lime Chicken Salad (page 185), ¾ cup cooked brown rice. 1 medium apple.

EVENING

Select any **one** of the following choices.
EACH SELECTION = APPROXIMATELY
300 CALORIES

- 1 serving Marinated Scallops (page 184), ⅓ cup brown rice. ½ cup fresh berries.
- 4 ounces Braised Steak (page 200), green salad with No Oil Dressing (page 189). ½ cup raspberries.
- 1 serving Alternative Cannelloni (page 214), green salad with lemon juice. ½ cup mixed sliced kiwifruit and strawberries.
- 1 Creamy Fish Roll with Dill Sauce (page 197), garden salad with 4 tablespoons Vinaigrette Dressing (page 189).
- 1 serving Baked Stuffed Fish (page 198), garden salad with No Oil Dressing (page 189), 1 cup sliced beets.
- ½ grilled chicken breast with 1 serving Pesto Sauce (page 193), garden salad with No Oil Dressing (page 189). 1 kiwifruit.
- 2 cups Quick Mexican Beans (page 209), garden salad

with No Oil Dressing (page 189). 1 slice dry rye toast. 1 medium sliced tomato.

- 2 cups Italian Noodle Soup (page 175), 4 whole wheat saltine crackers, green salad with No Oil Dressing (page 189). 1 medium pear.
- 1½ cups Minestrone Soup (page 173) with 2 slices dry whole grain toast, garden salad with No Oil Dressing (page 189). ½ cup unsweetened applesauce.
- 1 serving Chicken Kebabs (page 200), ½ cup cooked brown rice, green salad with 1 tablespoon raisins and lemon juice.
- 3.5 ounces lean grilled flank steak with 1 serving Chili Sauce (page 192), 1 cup carrots. 1 slice pineapple (approximately ¼ cup).
- 1 serving Butternut and Cashew Quiche (page 210), garden salad with lemon juice. 1 medium nectarine.

THYROID SHAPE EATING PLAN

Often it is the thyroid type of woman who comes to my clinic for advice because she is too thin and would love to put on some weight. She is often tired, stressed and experiencing mood swings.

The reason for this is the dominance of the thyroid gland, which keeps her metabolic rate so high that she burns calories very quickly.

The positive side to this is she has less risk of high cholesterol or obesity—provided her diet contains the correct balance of complex carbohydrates and protein.

The negative side is a tendency to continually stimulate her body with caffeine, alcohol, refined carbohydrates, sweets or nicotine. This overstimulates and eventually exhausts the thyroid gland. When this happens she may gain weight very quickly.

If you have become overweight and identify with this body type you should follow the weight-loss regime for thyroid shapes, which distributes calories evenly between breakfast, lunch and dinner. All meals are substantial and are designed to regulate energy fluctuations that are so common in thyroid types.

Never skip breakfast and avoid coffee in the mornings or you will be craving stimulants all day.

You must have some protein at every meal to stimulate your adrenal energy and to moderate your metabolism. Eat lots of whole grains, cereals and legumes to maintain stable blood sugar levels and eliminate mood swings and sweet cravings.

You tolerate dairy products well and the addition of natural low-fat yogurt with fruit will be more satisfying than eating fruit alone.

Late afternoon is your danger period when energy is at a low ebb. Avoid cake, chocolate or sweets as they will add empty calories and will not be as satisfying.

If you are not overweight and have not exhausted your thyroid gland, then forget the weight-loss program and follow the advice in our maintenance strategy—Step Two—to achieve optimum health.

STEP ONE:
WEIGHT LOSS FOR THE
THYROID BODY SHAPE

On waking have a large glass of water with a squeeze of lemon or lime juice.

THYROID GUIDELINES

FOOD GROUPS	DESIRABLE FOODS	UNDESIRABLE FOODS
Grains, cereal, bread and pasta	Whole grains such as brown rice, corn, rye, wheat, buckwheat, oats, millet and barley. Bread, crispbread, crackers, flour and pasta containing these whole grains.	Highly refined and bleached white flour products such as white bread, cookies and cakes. Avoid products made from bread or white cake flour.
Legumes	All beans, lentils and peas. Bean sprouts. Tofu.	
Meat, chicken, game and fish	Lean red meats. Chickens, turkeys and eggs. Fish and seafood.	Processed luncheon meats. Smoked and pickled meats and smoked seafood.
Dairy products	Most dairy products. Mild cheeses. Sheep and goats' milk and yogurt. Low-salt feta cheese.	Ripened cheeses. Chocolate.
Fruit and vegetables	All fresh and dried fruits, canned fruit in natural juice or water. A wide variety of fresh vegetables.	Fruit in sugar syrup, glazed fruit.

THYROID GUIDELINES (cont'd.)

FOOD GROUPS	DESIRABLE FOODS	UNDESIRABLE FOODS
Nuts and seeds	Unsalted raw nuts and seeds. Tahini and raw nut pastes.	Peanuts and salted nuts. Peanut butter. Coconut.
Fats and oils	Linseed, olive and canola oil. Butter or margarine.	Meat drippings, clarified butter and lard.
Beverages	Water: 6 to 12 glasses. Mineral water and seltzer. Cereal beverages (Postum, Ovaltine). Some herb teas. Decaffeinated coffee.	Carbonated soft drinks, cola drinks containing caffeine. Alcohol. Tannin-rich tea. Caffeine-rich coffee. Chocolate drinks.
Miscellaneous	Very small amounts of honey, sugar or molasses.	Refined sugars and products containing sugars. MSG. Artificial additives, preservatives and colors. Salt.

BREAKFAST

Select any one of the following choices.
**EACH SELECTION = APPROXIMATELY
300 CALORIES**

- 1 medium-sized poached egg, 6 ounces tomato juice or V8 vegetable juice cocktail, 1 slice whole grain toast, 1 tablespoon diet margarine. 1 serving of fresh fruit or juice.
- ½ cup low-fat 2% cottage cheese, 2 ounces dry whole grain bagel. 2 slices fresh pineapple (approximately ½ cup).
- ¼ cup part-skim ricotta cheese served on 2 slices whole grain toast. 4 ounces fresh orange juice.
- 2 small eggs beaten with 2 teaspoons low-fat calcium-enriched milk, mix in 3 chopped cherry tomatoes, 2 chopped mushrooms and fresh dill or coriander. Lightly cook and serve with 1 slice whole grain toast. 1 small serving of fruit or juice.
- 1 cup cooked rolled oats and 4 ounces low-fat 2% calcium-enriched milk, topped with 2 teaspoons LSA (page 263) and 2 teaspoons plain low-fat yogurt. 1 cup berries of your choice.
- 1 ounce breakfast cereal (page 242), 4 ounces low-fat 2% calcium-enriched milk or soy milk, add 2 teaspoons each LSA and plain low-fat yogurt, top with 1 medium sliced banana and 2 medium strawberries.
- ½ cup low-fat 2% plain yogurt blended with 4 ounces low-fat 2% calcium-enriched milk, ice cubes, ¾ cup fresh berries, 2 teaspoons LSA and 2 teaspoons wheat germ. 1 slice raisin bread.
- 1 ounce reduced-fat American cheese grilled on 2 slices whole grain toast. 6 ounces fresh orange juice.
- 2 slices rye bread topped with ¼ avocado, fresh lemon

or lime juice, black pepper and sprouts, if desired. 2 slices pineapple (approximately ½ cup).
- 2 Whole Wheat Pancakes (page 225) with 1 medium sliced banana and 2 medium strawberries. 1 tablespoon low-fat plain yogurt.

LUNCH

Select any **one** of the following choices.
EACH SELECTION = APPROXIMATELY 300 CALORIES

- 2 Ryvita crackers with 1 tablespoon Hummus (page 171), 3 ounces pink salmon, 1 medium sliced tomato, onion, cucumber, sprouts and freshly ground black pepper. 1 cup cantaloupe cubes.
- 1 whole grain roll (2 ounces) filled with 1 ounce chicken breast, 1 tablespoon light mayonnaise and unlimited salad greens with No Oil Dressing (page 189). 1 sliced kiwifruit and 5 strawberries.
- 2 slices rye bread with 1 ounce part-skim mozzarella cheese, sliced tomato, fresh basil or arugula leaves and freshly ground black pepper. 1 medium orange.
- ½ pita bread (1 ounce) filled with 1 Oven-Baked Falafel (page 207), 1 tablespoon Hummus (page 171) and unlimited salad greens and sprouts with No Oil Dressing (page 189). 1 large serving of fresh fruit or juice.
- 1 cup Minestrone Soup (page 173), 1 whole wheat English muffin, green salad vegetables with No Oil Dressing (page 189). Small bunch of grapes.
- 1 taco filled with 1 cup Quick Mexican Beans (page 209), shredded lettuce, sliced tomato and alfalfa sprouts topped with 1 tablespoon plain low-fat 2% plain yogurt and Chili Sauce (page 192). 1 large serving of fresh fruit or juice.

- 1 small baked potato with 1 serving Pesto Sauce (page 193), 1 serving Mushroom and Snow Pea Salad (page 183). ½ cup fruit salad.
- 3 ounces grilled white fish topped with lemon juice and chopped fennel (if desired), 1 serving Slimmers' Egg and Potato Salad (page 182), garden salad with No Oil Dressing (page 189). 2 slices fresh pineapple (approximately ½ cup).
- 2 ounces grilled lean meat with 1 serving Tomato Salsa (page 195), tossed green salad topped with lemon juice, 1 slice of rye bread. 1 kiwifruit.
- 1 serving Marinated Scallops (page 184) with ⅓ cup cooked brown rice. 1 cup watermelon balls.
- 1 serving Greek Salad (page 182), 2 Rye Krisps. ½ grapefruit.
- 1 cup pasta of your choice mixed with ¼ cup fresh chopped mushrooms, 2 halved cherry tomatoes, shallots, ¼ cup diced green pepper, ¼ cup snow peas and 2 ounces tuna in spring water (drained). You may add a little No Oil Dressing (page 189). ½ cup mixed melon balls.

EVENING

Select any **one** of the following choices.
**EACH SELECTION = APPROXIMATELY
400 CALORIES**

- 3 ounces lean grilled fillet steak with 2 tablespoons Blender Hollandaise (page 192), 1 small sweet potato, 1 cup steamed broccoli. 2 slices fresh pineapple (approximately ½ cup).
- 3.5 ounces lightly grilled veal rump with 1 serving Napolitana Sauce (page 216), 1 small baked potato with 1 tablespoon Mock Sour Cream Dressing (page 190), large

garden salad with lemon juice. 1 small serving of fresh fruit.

- 1 serving Baked Stuffed Fish (page 198), 1 small baked potato with 1 tablespoon Mock Sour Cream Dressing (page 190), green salad with 3 tablespoons Mustard Vinaigrette (page 188).
- ½ grilled chicken breast with 1 serving Tomato Salsa (page 195), 1 serving Slimmers' Egg and Potato Salad (page 182), 1 cup steamed green beans. 10 medium strawberries.
- 1 serving Butternut and Cashew Quiche (page 210), 1 cup sliced beets mixed with a little lemon juice, 1 grated carrot, large garden salad with 2 tablespoons Mustard Vinaigrette (page 188). 1 small serving of fresh fruit.
- 1 serving Fruit and Chicken Salad (page 186) with 1 cup cooked brown rice.
- 2 Cabbage Rolls (page 205), 1 medium baked potato and large garden salad with lemon juice. ½ cup fresh berries.
- 1 serving Low-Calorie Cannelloni (page 213), 1 small sweet potato, 1 cup steamed broccoli with 1 tablespoon roasted sunflower seeds. 1 small serving of fresh fruit.
- 2 Lentil Patties (page 208), 1 serving Spinach and Walnut Salad (page 181), 1 small baked potato. 1 cup cantaloupe cubes.
- 1 cup cooked spaghetti with Slimmers' Spaghetti Bolognese (page 212), green salad with lemon juice. 1 medium nectarine.
- 1 serving Pork and Pineapple Kebabs (page 199), 1 cup cauliflower, 1 serving Spinach and Walnut Salad (page 181).
- 3 ounces grilled white fish with 2 tablespoons Parsley Sauce (page 193), 1 serving Green Vegetable Plate with 2 tablespoons Dukkah (page 178). 1 medium apple.

CHAPTER THIRTEEN

STEP TWO: MAINTENANCE

CONGRATULATIONS ON YOUR SUCCESS!

You took up the challenge and you made the commitment to lose weight and change your body shape. You made a decision to be healthy and you have achieved the result.

In order to do it, you had to become more active, change your attitude, your eating habits and your cooking methods. Change never comes easily but **you found your power and you took control**. You made the right choices. *You* did it!

Put the book down for a moment and go take a long look at yourself in the mirror. Look at yourself with pride and know that the person you see is worthy of compliments.

You must never allow anybody or anything to undermine your self-esteem again.

> **Remember that your achievements are proof of your inner strength and your ability to do things for yourself.**

THE TRANSITION TO WEIGHT MAINTENANCE

Once you have achieved a weight that (a) pleases you and (b) falls within the healthy weight range (see Chapter Three), you are ready to start our Weight Maintenance Program Step Two. Refer to the table on page 25 to estimate your caloric intake to maintain your current desired weight.

Do not start at that caloric level immediately because you are a unique individual and your level for weight maintenance may not perfectly match that in the table. It is only to be used as a general guideline.

To identify *your* ideal level for weight maintenance you must increase your caloric intake gradually. This will ensure that you make a smooth transition between weight loss and weight maintenance.

Begin by increasing your daily caloric intake by 200 calories for the first week of maintenance.

This may be achieved simply by adding some extra servings of fruit and complex carbohydrates. For example:

2 additional servings of fruit and an extra serving of bread.

or

2 additional servings of fruit and an extra ½ cup of rice.

or

2 additional servings of fruit and an extra small baked potato.

Gradually increase your daily intake week by week until you stop losing weight and your body weight stabilizes.

At this point you will note your ideal weight for your Maintenance level. It is natural for your weight to fluctuate slightly, so add and subtract 4 to 5 pounds from this and you now have a comfortable weight range that you will easily stay within.

As soon as you go above your 4- to 5-pound margin then

go back to Step One—the Body-Shaping Diet weight-loss program, until you are back at your ideal weight and then stick to your Maintenance Program—Step Two.

SUCCESSFUL WEIGHT MAINTENANCE

Remember that the Body-Shaping Diet allowed you to lose your weight gradually, which makes it much easier to maintain. Be confident; you have worked hard to change your metabolism and you have succeeded. You no longer have to put so much energy into controlling your weight.

As a guideline, I have included a range of sample menus for each body shape that are calculated at 1400 calories each day. You may need to make adjustments to this, according to your ideal caloric level, to achieve successful maintenance. Choose freely from our recipe section, which also has some delicious sweets for special occasions.

The increase in calories in Step Two allows you the freedom to once again look forward to dinner parties or restaurant meals and even have several courses without fear of weight gain. You can relax a little on birthdays and at other celebrations as long as they are special occasions and not daily occurrences.

Remember, it's what you do 95 percent of the time that counts.

Never go back to the negative patterns that caused you to be unhealthy and overweight.

To maintain optimum health and achieve successful weight maintenance you should continue your exercise program. Even though it may have seemed a chore at first, you know that it helped your weight loss, toned your body and increased your fitness level.

By now you will have found a sport or exercise routine that you look forward to and will continue to enjoy.

I recommend that you weigh yourself once a week at

the same time of day. Self-monitoring of your weight will make it easier to maintain.

If you find your weight is creeping back due to a lapse in routine, return to Step One and increase your exercise. Be sure to eliminate any foods that are high in fat or sugar.

If you are feeling a lack of confidence and self-control, be sure to remind yourself of your achievements and ability. Contact a reliable friend or psychologist if you need help with a difficult situation.

I encourage you to shop wisely and to continue with your new cooking methods. By now your new habits will have become routine. If some of your old habits start creeping back, think about why you changed them and recommit yourself.

Follow the guidelines for your body shape (beginning on page 104), maintain your exercise program and enjoy good health.

STEP TWO: MAINTENANCE FOR THE ANDROID BODY SHAPE

On waking have a large glass of water with a squeeze of lemon or lime juice.

BREAKFAST

Select any one of the following choices
EACH SELECTION = APPROXIMATELY 350 CALORIES

- 1 Whole Wheat Pancake (page 225), 1½ cups fresh berries, 8 ounces plain low-fat yogurt, 2 teaspoons LSA (page 263). Cup of herbal tea.

- 1 ounce breakfast cereal (page 242), 4 ounces low-fat 2% calcium-enriched milk, soy milk or Rice Dream milk, ½ tablespoon each lecithin and LSA, 6 medium strawberries. 1 slice whole grain toast with 1 teaspoon spreadable fruit.
- 2 slices dry whole grain toast with ½ cup low-fat 2% cottage cheese, sliced tomato and alfalfa sprouts, if desired. 6 ounces fresh orange juice.
- 1 cup cooked rolled oats with 4 ounces low-fat 2% calcium-enriched milk, soy milk or Rice Dream milk and ½ sliced banana and 3 strawberries, 2 teaspoons each LSA (page 263) and wheat germ. Cup of herbal tea.
- 1 Whole Wheat Pancake (page 225), ½ cup part-skim ricotta cheese. 1 cup cantaloupe cubes, 4 ounces fresh orange juice.
- 2 slices dry whole grain toast with 2 ounces fresh turkey breast. 1 large apple.
- ½ cup fresh fruit of your choice blended with 4 ounces low-fat 2% calcium-enriched milk, soy milk or Rice Dream milk, ice cubes and ½ tablespoon lecithin and wheat germ. 2 slices raisin bread.
- 1 poached or boiled egg with Blender Hollandaise (page 192) and fresh parsley, if desired, on 2 slices dry whole grain toast served with 1 tablespoon diet margarine. 4 ounces fresh orange juice.
- 2 Banana and Pecan Muffins (page 227). Cup dandelion beverage.
- 2 slices whole grain toast spread with 2 ounces reduced-fat American cheese. ¾ cup grapes.
- 1 toasted whole wheat English muffin topped with 4 teaspoons spreadable fruit. 1 medium banana.
- 2 slices dry whole grain toast with ½ avocado, fresh tomato slices, chopped chives and freshly ground black pepper. 2 slices pineapple (approximately ½ cup).

LUNCH

Select any **one** of the following choices.
**EACH SELECTION = APPROXIMATELY
450 CALORIES**

- ½ cup Guacamole (page 171), at least 2 cups mixed fresh raw vegetables to dip (e.g. radish, fennel, carrot, zucchini, green pepper, celery and broccoli florets). 1 slice pumpernickel with 1 tablespoon Hummus (page 171). 1 medium pear.
- 1 pita bread (2 ounces) with 2 Oven-Baked Falafel (page 207), lettuce, 1 tablespoon each of Hummus (page 171) and Tabbouli Salad (page 176). 1 medium banana.
- Whole wheat roll (2 ounces) with a Lentil Patty (page 208), fresh green salad, tomato and ¼ medium avocado. 8 ounces fresh orange juice.
- 2 cups Italian Noodle Soup (page 175), green salad with No Oil Dressing (page 189). 2 slices whole grain bread. 1 large serving fresh fruit.
- 3.5 ounces pink salmon and ½ cup low-fat 2% cottage cheese, garden salad, 1 cup sliced beets. 2 Ryvita wheat crackers. 1 nectarine.
- 2 slices dry whole grain toast with ½ cup part-skim ricotta cheese and 1 medium fresh tomato, onion and fresh basil with 1 tablespoon Vinaigrette Dressing (page 189). 3 slices fresh pineapple (approximately ⅔ cup).
- 1 cup cooked pasta spirals mixed with 2.5 ounces chopped cooked chicken, 4 chopped sun-dried tomatoes, 1 teaspoon olive oil, 1 tablespoon pine nuts and 1 cup chopped raw mushrooms, shallots, celery, radish, fennel, broccoli, bean sprouts mixed together, with fresh parsley and mint, if desired. 1 small orange.
- Mixed Bean and Rice Salad (page 179). 1 cup cantaloupe cubes.
- 2 Quick Curried Eggs (page 211), garden salad with

No Oil Dressing (page 189), 1 slice rye bread with 1 tablespoon tahini. 10 strawberries.

- 1 serving Fresh Asparagus Vinaigrette (page 177), 1 medium baked potato with 1 tablespoon Mock Sour Cream Dressing (page 190), 1 medium corn on the cob, 2 Ryvita sesame crackers. 1 medium peach.
- 1 serving Low-Calorie Cannelloni (page 213), 1 serving Beet and Watercress Salad (page 180), ½ cup zucchini, 1 small corn on the cob. 1 slice rye bread. 1 small serving of fresh fruit or juice.
- 1½ cups Squash Soup (page 174), 2 slices rye bread. 1 serving Spinach and Walnut Salad (page 181). 1 cup watermelon balls.

EVENING

Select any **one** of the following choices.
**EACH SELECTION = APPROXIMATELY
600 CALORIES**

- 3.5 ounces grilled white fish with 1 serving Florentine Sauce (page 194), 1 serving Tomato Salsa (page 195), 1 small baked potato with 2 teaspoons Mock Sour Cream Dressing (page 190), 1 medium corn on the cob, ½ cup green beans, 3 brussels sprouts. ½ cup fruit salad.
- 1 serving Tuna Bake (page 222), 1 cup sliced beets, green salad with No Oil Dressing (page 189). 1 small serving of fresh fruit.
- 1 serving Green Vegetable Plate with 2 tablespoons Dukkah (page 178), 1 cup Dahl (page 210), 1 cup cooked brown rice. Banana Cream (page 218) with 1 cup mixed berries.
- 2 small taco shells filled with 1 cup Quick Mexican Beans (page 209), 1 cup mixed fresh chopped tomato,

shredded lettuce, alfalfa sprouts, 1 tablespoon plain low-fat yogurt and ½ cup Chili Sauce (page 192). 1 large corn on the cob. 1 serving Lemon Self-Saucing Pudding (page 232).

- 1½ cups Squash Soup (page 174), Lentil Patty (page 208) on a whole wheat roll (2 ounces) with ¼ avocado, salad greens and sprouts, ½ cup Chili Sauce (page 192). 2 slices fresh pineapple (approximately ½ cup).

- 4 ounces Braised Steak (page 200), ½ cup cooked brown rice, garden salad with 3 tablespoons dressing of your choice. 1 serving Fresh Fruit Sorbet (page 231).

- 1 cup Minestrone Soup (page 173), 1 serving Alternative Cannelloni (page 214), 4 ounces sweet potato, 1 cup carrots, ½ cup cauliflower, ½ cup lightly cooked mushrooms. 1 small serving of fresh fruit.

- 7 ounces Baked Stuffed Fish (page 198), 1 medium baked potato with 1 tablespoon Mock Sour Cream Dressing (page 190), 3 Stuffed Mushroom Caps (page 169), ½ cup cabbage, ½ cup green beans. 1 slice rye bread.

- 2 cups cooked spaghetti with 2 servings Pesto Sauce (page 193), garden salad with No Oil Dressing (page 189). 2 cups raspberries and strawberries.

- 1 serving Avocado and Chicken in Filo (page 204), ½ cup mashed potato with finely chopped onion and parsley, 1 cup carrots, 2 brussels sprouts. 1 small serving of fresh fruit.

- Kidney Bean Bake (recipe page 206), 1 small baked potato, 1 serving Carrot and Raisin Salad (recipe page 181), 1 serving Green Vegetable Plate with 1 tablespoon Dukkah (page 178). 1 small serving of fresh fruit.

- 1 cup Zucchini Soup (page 174) and 2 slices toasted rye bread. 2 Cabbage Rolls (page 205), ½ cup peas and 1 cup green beans. 1 serving Fresh Fruit Sorbet (page 231).

STEP TWO:
MAINTENANCE FOR THE
GYNECOID BODY SHAPE

On waking have a large glass of water with a squeeze of lemon or lime juice.

BREAKFAST

Select any **one** of the following choices.
EACH SELECTION = APPROXIMATELY 350 CALORIES

- 1 cup cooked brown rice, 4 ounces low-fat 2% calcium-enriched milk or soy milk, 2 teaspoons wheat germ, ½ banana and 6 small or 3 large strawberries.
- ¾ cup cooked rolled oats, 4 ounces low-fat 2% calcium-enriched milk, skim milk, or low-fat soy milk, sprinkled with cinnamon, nutmeg or vanilla, 1 small banana. 1 slice raisin toast. Cup of herbal tea.
- 1 poached or boiled egg, 1 tablespoon diet margarine with fresh parsley, 2 slices whole grain toast. Serve with tomato and snow pea sprouts. 4 ounces fresh orange juice.
- Fruit shake: your choice of small piece of fruit blended with 8 ounces low-fat 2% calcium-enriched milk or soy milk, ice cubes and ½ tablespoon each LSA (page 263) and wheat germ. 2 slices raisin bread.
- 2 slices whole grain toast topped with ⅓ avocado, squeeze of lemon or lime juice and freshly ground black pepper. 1 medium banana. Cup of herbal tea.
- 1 ounce breakfast cereal (page 242), 4 ounces low-fat

2% calcium-enriched milk or soy milk, 2 teaspoons wheat germ, ½ cup fresh berries. 1 slice rye toast with 2 teaspoons tahini. Cup of dandelion beverage.

- 2 Whole Wheat Pancakes (page 225) with ½ sliced banana, 5 large strawberries and 1 serving Vanilla Yogurt Sauce (page 236). Cup of herbal tea.
- 1 boiled egg with 1 slice rye toast, 2 Blueberry Muffins (page 227). Cup of herbal tea.
- 1 toasted whole wheat English muffin topped with ¼ cup part-skim ricotta cheese, 1 medium banana.
- 2 slices whole grain toast, 4 ounces fresh turkey breast. 1 cup cantaloupe cubes.

LUNCH

Select any **one** of the following choices.
**EACH SELECTION = APPROXIMATELY
450 CALORIES**

- 3.5 ounces pink salmon, 2 halves Deviled Eggs (page 170), sliced tomato, 1 cup sliced beets and unlimited green salad with No Oil Dressing (page 189). 1 slice rye bread. 3 slices fresh pineapple (approximately ⅔ cup).
- ½ avocado and alfalfa sprouts sandwich on 2 slices whole grain bread thinly spread with 1 tablespoon Hummus (page 171). 8-ounce carton nonfat sugar-free fruit yogurt.
- Whole wheat roll (2 ounces) with 1 sliced hard-boiled egg, lettuce, sprouts, cucumber and 1 teaspoon light mayonnaise. 1 Apple and Oat Bran Muffin (page 226). ½ cup unsweetened canned peaches.
- 1 cup Squash Soup (page 174), 1 whole wheat roll (2 ounces), garden salad with 1 tablespoon dressing of your choice. 1 medium banana.
- Omelet made from 2 eggs and 1 tablespoon low-fat 2%

milk, 5 cherry tomatoes, ½ cup chopped fresh mushrooms, chives or shallots and parsley, paprika, if desired. 2 slices whole wheat toast. 1 medium pear.

- 1.5 ounces sardines in spring water (drained), ¼ cup 2% milkfat cottage cheese, garden salad with 1 tablespoon dressing of your choice. 1 whole wheat roll (2 ounces). 8 ounces fresh orange juice.

- 1 pita bread (2 ounces) with 2 Oven-Baked Falafel (page 207), lettuce, 1 tablespoon each Hummus (page 171) and Tabbouli Salad (page 176). 1 medium banana.

- ½ grilled chicken breast with 1 serving Florentine Sauce (page 194), garden salad and 4 tablespoons Mustard Vinaigrette (page 188), 1 cup sliced beets mixed with lemon juice. 4 slices fresh pineapple (approximately 1 cup).

- 3.5 ounces grilled fish with 2 tablespoons Blender Hollandaise (page 192) and fresh parsley, 3 Stuffed Mushroom Caps (page 169), 1 small baked potato with 2 teaspoons Mock Sour Cream Dressing (page 190), garden salad with No Oil Dressing (page 189). 1 cup cantaloupe cubes.

- 1 serving Pork and Pineapple Kebabs (page 199), ½ cup sliced beets, 1 small corn on the cob, 1 serving Green Bean and Apple Salad (page 180). 1 slice rye bread.

- 1 cup cooked pasta with 1 serving Pesto Sauce (page 193), garden salad with 2 tablespoons Vinaigrette Dressing (page 189), 1 serving Carrot and Raisin Salad (page 181). 1 kiwifruit.

- 1 serving Mixed Bean and Rice Salad (page 179), ½ cup unsweetened applesauce.

EVENING

Select any **one** of the following choices.
**EACH SELECTION = APPROXIMATELY
600 CALORIES**

- 3.5 ounces lean, grilled flank steak, 1 serving Tomato Salsa (page 195), 1 small sweet potato, 1 cup cauliflower, 1 medium corn on the cob, 1 cup fresh green beans. Minted Pineapple Sorbet (page 229).
- ½ grilled chicken breast topped with fresh lime juice, chopped fresh ginger and tarragon. 1 medium baked potato with 2 tablespoons Mock Sour Cream Dressing (page 190). 1 cup sliced beets, 1 serving Spinach and Walnut Salad (page 181), 1½ cups cantaloupe cubes. Iced Peach Treat (page 228).
- 1 serving Irish Stew (page 201), 2 slices whole grain toast. 1 small orange.
- 6 ounces Tandoori Fish (page 196), 1 cup cooked brown rice, 1 serving Minted Tomato Salsa (page 195), 1 cup green beans, 3 brussels sprouts. Your choice of ½ cup mixed fresh fruit.
- 1 cup Minestrone Soup (page 173) with 1 slice rye bread, 1 serving Low-Calorie Cannelloni (page 213), 1 medium corn on the cob, ½ cup carrots and unlimited green salad with No Oil Dressing (page 189). 1 small serving of fresh fruit.
- 1 serving Chicken and Vegetable Hot Pot (page 202) with 1 small whole wheat dinner roll, 1 serving Beet and Watercress Salad (page 180). 1 serving Strawberry-Melon Mousse (page 230).
- 1 serving Butternut and Cashew Quiche (page 210), 1 serving Greek Salad (page 182). 1 cup fruit salad.
- 2 Cabbage Rolls (page 205), 1 small baked potato, 1 cup carrots, ½ cup peas. 1 serving Minted Pineapple Sorbet (page 229).

- 1 serving Lamb and Fruit Kebabs (page 199), 1 small baked potato with 2 tablespoons Mock Sour Cream Dressing (page 190), 1 serving Tomato Salsa (page 195), 1 serving Spinach and Walnut Salad (page 181).
- 2 cups cooked spaghetti with 1 serving Pesto Sauce (page 193), garden salad with 2 carrot sticks and 1 tablespoon Vinaigrette Dressing (page 189). Poached pear half with 2 tablespoons Almond Custard Cream (page 235).
- 7 ounces Baked Stuffed Fish (page 198), 1 small sweet potato, 1 cup cauliflower, 1 cup green beans. ½ cup Berry Delicious (page 229).
- 1 serving Chicken in a Parcel (page 221), 1¼ cups Pasta Salad (page 179). 1 small serving fresh fruit of your choice.

STEP TWO:
MAINTENANCE FOR THE
LYMPHATIC BODY SHAPE

On waking have a large glass of water with a squeeze of lemon or lime juice.

BREAKFAST

Select any **one** of the following choices.
**EACH SELECTION = APPROXIMATELY
450 CALORIES**

- 1 ounce breakfast cereal (page 242) with 8 ounces soy milk or Rice Dream milk, 2 teaspoons oat bran and 1 tablespoon mixed roasted sesame and sunflower seeds. 3 Flapjacks (page 236), ½ banana.

- 1 cup cooked oats with 4 ounces Rice Dream milk or soy milk. ½ cup fresh berries and 2 teaspoons LSA (page 263). 1 slice whole grain toast with 2 ounces fresh turkey breast.
- 1 kiwifruit blended with 8 ounces soy milk or Rice Dream milk, ice cubes and ½ tablespoon each lecithin, wheat germ and oat bran. 1 Apple and Oat Bran Muffin (page 226) served with 1 teaspoon tahini. Cup of herbal tea.
- 2 slices dry whole grain toast with ½ medium-sized avocado topped with fresh lime or lemon juice and black pepper. 8 ounces fresh orange juice.
- 2 poached eggs, 2 slices dry whole grain toast, served with 2 tablespoons diet margarine. 1 cup cantaloupe cubes.
- 2 slices dry whole grain toast with 2 ounces fresh turkey breast. 1 medium pear.
- 3 Whole Wheat Pancakes (page 225) with 1 banana and ¾ cup mixed berries. Cup of herbal tea.
- 8 ounces soy milk, 2 Apple and Oat Bran Muffins (page 226). 1 large orange. Cup of herbal tea.
- 1 toasted whole wheat English muffin topped with 1 cup Dahl (page 210) and fresh parsley, if desired. 1 small serving of fruit or juice.
- 2 slices dry toasted rye bread with 4 ounces fresh turkey breast. 6 ounces apple juice.

LUNCH

Select any **one** of the following choices.
**EACH SELECTION = APPROXIMATELY
550 CALORIES**

- 2 Quick Curried Eggs (page 211), 6 carrot sticks, garden

salad and No Oil Dressing (page 189), 2 slices dry whole grain toast. 1 large apple.

- 3.5 ounces pink salmon (drained), 1 medium potato, 1 cup sliced beets, garden salad with 2 tablespoons Hazelnut Dressing (page 190). 2 slices fresh pineapple and 1 kiwifruit.

- 3.5 ounces fresh baked or grilled white fish with 1 serving Pesto Sauce (page 193), 1 serving Tomato Salsa (page 195), 1 small potato, 1 serving Mushroom and Snow Pea Salad (page 183). ½ cup mixed berries.

- 3 ounces lean grilled London broil with 1 serving Mustard Sauce (page 194), 1 cup zucchini, 1 cup carrots. Iced Peach Treat (page 228) or 2 cups cantaloupe cubes.

- Lentil Patty (page 208) on whole wheat roll (2 ounces), garden salad with 2 tablespoons Raspberry Vinaigrette (page 191) and Chili Sauce (page 192). 1 large serving of fresh fruit or juice of your choice.

- 1 serving Tuna Bake (page 222), green salad with No Oil Dressing (page 189). 1 cup cantaloupe cubes.

- 1 pita bread (2 ounces) filled with 2 Oven-Baked Falafel (page 207), 1½ tablespoons Hummus (page 171), ¼ avocado, garden salad with lemon juice. 8 ounces fresh orange juice.

- 1 serving Mixed Bean and Rice Salad (page 179). 1 slice pumpernickel with 1 teaspoon tahini. 1 small serving of fresh fruit or juice.

- ½ grilled chicken breast with Chili Sauce (page 192), garden salad with fresh lemon juice, 1 large corn on the cob. 1 serving Baked Rice Pudding (page 230) with 1 medium banana.

- 2 cups cooked spaghetti with 2 servings Pesto Sauce (page 193) and garden salad with fresh lemon juice. 1 medium peach.

- 2 cups Italian Noodle Soup (page 175), 1 whole wheat English muffin, 1 serving Green Vegetable Plate with 2

tablespoons Dukkah (page 178). 1 small serving of fresh
fruit of your choice.
- 1 serving Fruit and Chicken Salad (page 186), 1 cup
cooked brown rice, 1 cup Cucumber Salad (page 186).
1 medium apple.

EVENING

Select any **one** of the following choices.
EACH SELECTION = APPROXIMATELY
400 CALORIES

- 1 serving Marinated Scallops (page 184) with ½ cup
cooked brown rice. 1 cup fresh berries.
- 3 ounces Braised Steak (page 200), 1 small corn on the
cob, garden salad with 1 tablespoon Vinaigrette Dressing
(page 189). 1 serving Fresh Fruit Sorbet (page 221).
- 1 serving Alternative Cannelloni (page 214), 1 small
sweet potato, ½ cup carrots, ½ cup green beans. 1 kiwifruit.
- Slimmers' Spaghetti Bolognese (page 212) with 1 cup
cooked pasta, garden salad with lemon juice. 10 medium
strawberries.
- 7 ounces Baked Stuffed Fish (page 198), 1 small baked
potato, garden salad with No Oil Dressing (page 189),
1 cup sliced beets. 1 medium peach.
- ½ grilled chicken breast with 1 serving Pesto Sauce
(page 193), 1 small corn on the cob, 3 broccoli florets.
1 small serving of fruit of your choice.
- 1½ cups Quick Mexican Beans (page 209), garden salad
with No Oil Dressing (page 189). 1 serving Babaganouj
(page 172), 1 tablespoon Hummus (page 171), ½ pita
bread. 1 cup watermelon balls.
- 2 cups Italian Noodle Soup (page 175), 2 slices toasted

rye bread, 2 servings Beet and Watercress Salad (page 180). 1 serving Poached Pears (page 234).

- 1 serving Lime Chicken Salad (page 185) with ¾ cup cooked brown rice. 1 small serving of fresh fruit of your choice.
- 1 serving Pork and Pineapple Kebabs (page 199), 1 small corn on the cob, 1 serving sliced Beet and Watercress Salad (page 180).
- 3.5 ounces lean grilled steak with Chili Sauce (page 192), ½ cup carrots, 4 brussels sprouts. 1 serving Fresh Fruit Sorbet (page 231).
- 1 serving Butternut and Cashew Quiche (page 210), 1 serving Green Bean and Apple Salad (page 180), 1 small baked potato. 5 medium strawberries.

STEP TWO:
MAINTENANCE FOR THE
THYROID BODY SHAPE

On waking have a large glass of water with a squeeze of lemon or lime juice.

BREAKFAST

Select any **one** of the following choices.
**EACH SELECTION = APPROXIMATELY
400 CALORIES**

- 2 poached eggs with 2 tablespoons Blender Hollandaise (page 192) and freshly chopped parsley, 2 slices whole grain toast served with fresh tomato and alfalfa or snow pea sprouts, if desired. 4 ounces fresh orange juice.

- 2 ounces reduced-fat American cheese, 2 slices rye toast. 1 medium pear.
- 2 slices whole grain toast spread with ½ cup part-skim ricotta cheese. 1 medium apple.
- 2-egg omelet beaten with 2 tablespoons low-fat 2% calcium-enriched milk, mix in 3 chopped cherry tomatoes and ½ cup chopped mushrooms and fresh dill or coriander, lightly cook in pan coated with nonstick cooking spray. Serve with 2 slices whole grain toast. 1 small serving of fruit or juice of your choice.
- 1 cup cooked rolled oats, 4 ounces low-fat 2% calcium-enriched milk, topped with 2 teaspoons LSA (page 263) and 2 teaspoons plain low-fat yogurt, ½ banana. 1 Blueberry Muffin (page 227). Cup of herbal tea.
- ½ cup cooked fresh mushrooms served on 1 whole wheat English muffin spread with 1 tablespoon Hummus (page 171), top with fresh chopped parsley if desired, 4 ounces low-fat 2% calcium-enriched milk blended with 1 small banana and flavored with vanilla and ground nutmeg.
- 1 ounce breakfast cereal (page 242), 4 ounces low-fat 2% calcium-enriched milk or soy milk, add 2 teaspoons each LSA (page 263) and plain low-fat yogurt, top with 2 medium fresh strawberries and ½ banana. 1 slice whole grain toast with 2 teaspoons tahini. Cup of herbal tea.
- 4 ounces plain low-fat yogurt blended with 4 ounces low-fat 2% calcium-enriched milk, ice cubes, 1 cup fresh berries, 2 teaspoons LSA (page 263) and 2 teaspoons wheat germ. 1 Banana and Pecan Muffin (page 227).
- 1 ounce reduced-fat American cheese grilled on 2 slices whole grain toast, topped with ¼ cup chopped green pepper, mushroom and chives, if desired. 4 ounces fresh orange juice. 1 medium pear.
- 2 slices rye toast with ¼ avocado, fresh lemon juice, black pepper and sprouts. 1 small pear. 8 ounces low-fat 2% calcium-enriched milk.
- 2 Whole Wheat Pancakes (page 225) with 1 medium

sliced banana, 7 medium strawberries, 1 serving Vanilla Yogurt Sauce (page 236).
- 1 cup cooked barley with 4 ounces low-fat 2% calcium-enriched milk, 1 tablespoon plain low-fat yogurt, 2 teaspoons LSA (page 263), 1½ tablespoons raisins, 2 teaspoons wheat germ.

LUNCH

Select any **one** of the following choices.
EACH SELECTION = APPROXIMATELY
450 CALORIES

- 2 slices rye toast with 1 tablespoon Hummus (page 171), 3.5 ounces pink salmon, 1 medium sliced tomato, onion, cucumber, sprouts and freshly ground black pepper. 1 cup cantaloupe.
- 1 whole wheat roll (2 ounces) filled with 3 ounces chicken, 1 tablespoon light mayonnaise, ¼ avocado and unlimited salad with No Oil Dressing (page 189). ½ cup sliced kiwifruit and strawberries.
- 1 serving Greek Salad (page 182), 1 serving Babaganouj (page 172), ½ pita bread. 1 medium peach.
- 1 pita bread (1 ounce) with 2 Oven-Baked Falafel (page 207), 1 tablespoon Hummus (page 171) and ½ cup Tabbouli Salad (page 176), lettuce and sprouts. 1 small serving of fresh fruit or juice.
- 2 cups Italian Noodle Soup (page 175), 1 whole wheat English muffin, 3 spears Fresh Asparagus Vinaigrette (page 177). Small bunch of grapes.
- 2 tacos filled with 1 cup Quick Mexican Beans (page 209), 1 ounce grated low-fat cheese, shredded lettuce, sliced tomato, alfalfa sprouts and topped with 2 tablespoons plain low-fat yogurt and Chili Sauce (page 192). 1 large serving of fresh fruit or juice.

- 1 serving Chickpea Curry (page 220), ½ cup brown rice, Beet and Watercress Salad (page 180). ½ cup fruit salad.
- 3.5 ounces grilled white fish topped with 2 servings Egg Sauce (page 194), garden salad with No Oil Dressing (page 189), 1 serving Carrot and Raisin Salad (page 181). 2 slices fresh pineapple (approximately ½ cup).
- 3.5 ounces grilled lean beef with 1 serving Tomato Salsa (page 195), 1 small baked potato with 1 tablespoon Mock Sour Cream Dressing (page 190), green salad vegetables topped with lemon juice and 1 teaspoon roasted sesame seeds. 1 kiwifruit.
- 4 ounces Marinated Scallops (page 184) with ¾ cup cooked brown rice. ½ cup Cucumber Salad (page 186). 1 small orange.
- 1 serving Salmon Mornay (page 223), green salad with lemon juice. 1 small fresh fruit of your choice.
- 1 serving Mixed Bean and Rice Salad (page 179). 1 cup mixed cantaloupe, watermelon and honeydew balls.

EVENING

Select any **one** of the following choices.
EACH SELECTION = APPROXIMATELY 550 CALORIES

- 1 cup cooked pasta with 1 serving Eggplant and Napolitana Sauce (page 216). 2 cups fresh pineapple and strawberries.
- 4 ounces Caribbean Chicken (page 220), ¼ cup cooked rice, 1 serving Green Vegetable Plate with 2 tablespoons Dukkah (page 178). 1 serving Fresh Fruit Sorbet (page 231).
- 1 serving Tuna Bake (page 222), green salad with No Oil Dressing (page 189). 1 small fresh fruit of your choice.

- 1 serving Chicken in a Parcel (page 221), ¾ cup Slimmers' Egg and Potato Salad (page 182), 1 cup steamed broccoli, green beans and snow peas. ½ cup sliced kiwifruit and strawberries.
- 1 serving Butternut and Cashew Quiche (page 210), 1 cup steamed spinach mixed with a little lemon juice, 1 cup corn, garden salad with 3 tablespoons Mustard Vinaigrette (page 188). 1 cup melon balls.
- 1 serving Seafood Salad (page 184) with ½ cup cooked brown rice. ½ cup Berry Delicious (page 229).
- 2 Cabbage Rolls (page 205), 1 medium baked potato, large garden salad with lemon juice. 1 serving Apple Crumble (page 233) with 2 tablespoons Almond Custard Cream (page 235).
- 1 serving Irish Stew (page 201), ½ cup brown rice, green salad with No Oil Dressing (page 189). 1 serving Fresh Fruit Sorbet (page 178).
- 2 Lentil Patties (page 208), 1 small baked potato with 1 serving Pesto Sauce (page 193), 1 serving Spinach and Walnut Salad (page 181). Medium bunch of grapes (approximately 1½ cups).
- 1 cup cooked spaghetti with 1 serving Authentic Bolognese Sauce (page 223), green salad with lemon juice. 1 serving Fresh Fruit Sorbet (page 231).
- 1 serving Lamb and Fruit Kebabs (page 199), ½ cup cooked brown rice, 1 serving Spinach and Walnut Salad (page 181).
- 5 ounces grilled white fish with 1 serving Parsley Sauce (page 193), ½ cup mashed potatoes, ½ cup carrots. 1 serving Minted Pineapple Sorbet (page 229).

CHAPTER FOURTEEN

HELPFUL HERBAL TEAS

ANDROID	GYNECOID	LYMPHATIC	THYROID
Black cohosh	Red clover	Red bush tea	Valerian
Raspberry leaf	Fennel	Lemongrass	Chamomile
Blue flag	Parsley	Blue flag	Licorice root*
Rosemary	Lemongrass	Rose hip	Fenugreek
Shepherd's purse	Hibiscus	Hibiscus	Nettle
Sarsaparilla	Chamomile	Dandelion	Rosemary
Dandelion	Peppermint	Nettle	Fennel
Lemon balm	Nettle	Ginger	Alfalfa
Ginger	Red bush tea	Fennel	Lemon balm
Cinnamon	Dandelion	Parsley	Passion flower

*LICORICE ROOT. This herb, like all herbs, should not be taken during pregnancy or if you have high blood pressure.

PREPARATION

All of the herbal teas listed can be purchased at health food stores or supermarkets. Perhaps you have them in your garden.

You may wish to combine some of the bland herbs with an aromatic one to improve the flavor of the tea. Some good combinations are:

> CHAMOMILE and PEPPERMINT
> RASPBERRY LEAF and GINGER
> NETTLE and FENNEL
> ALFALFA and ROSEMARY

You will be able to buy some of the herbs already packaged in tea bags for your convenience. For the other herbs follow the instructions given below.

The flowers and leaves of herbs are prepared by making a tea. Allow ½ ounce or ½ cup of the dried herb to 1 cup of boiled water. Prepare the tea in a glass or ceramic teapot with a tight-fitting lid. Let the infusion steep for 10 to 15 minutes, then strain and drink.

If you are using the dried root, seeds, bark or woody parts of a plant, you will need to make a decoction. This is made by adding ½ ounce or ½ cup of the dried herb to 1 cup of cold water in a glass or enamel saucepan. Let the mixture soak for 10 minutes, then cover and bring to a boil. Reduce the heat and simmer for 15 minutes. Remove from the heat and let steep a further 10 minutes. Strain and drink warm.

DOSAGE

A cupful should be taken warm, not hot, three times a day.

ANDROID SHAPE— HERBAL TEAS

For your body type it is essential that you use herbs that will rebalance your adrenal glands and also include some with estrogenic properties to restore the balance of female hormones in your body.

One of the best herbal teas for this purpose is **black cohosh**. It is a herb that is good for estrogen insufficiency.

Raspberry leaf tea is also estrogenic, nutritive and is a tonic to your reproductive system.

Blue flag is a herb that suits your body type well. Its main action is on the liver and skin and it is specific for eruptive skin conditions. Your body type can be prone to acne and drinking this herb as a tea will help you to cleanse from the inside.

Rosemary is a calming herb that is specific for neuralgia or migraine headaches. If you don't like it as a tea then use it as a culinary herb to serve with potato or chicken dishes.

Shepherd's purse regulates your menstrual flow and will help prevent spotting between periods. You will probably find it growing in your backyard or between cracks in paths. It might be wiser to buy the dried plant, unless you are certain that no poisons have been sprayed around and that pets have not been there first.

Sarsaparilla is a tonic herb that can improve your libido. It is an excellent treatment for rheumatism and gout because it assists in the elimination of urea or uric acid. You may be familiar with this herb, as it is used as a flavoring agent in soft drinks.

Dandelion is a coffee substitute that is a tonic to the liver and kidneys. Its action on the liver will assist your body's ability to metabolize cholesterol.

Lemon balm is a pleasant-tasting diaphoretic tea. This means it will help eliminate toxins via the skin. Your body type often has a problem with unhealthy skin and this herb will help.

Ginger and cinnamon are stimulant herbs that aid digestion and prevent cramping. When taken as a tea, they are great for abdominal cramps and ovarian or uterine pain.

GYNECOID SHAPE— HERBAL TEAS

I have carefully chosen teas that will not overstimulate your ovaries. I have picked **red clover** as a tonic to your reproductive system. Try to have at least one cupful of tea made from this herb each day.

Fennel is slightly estrogenic; however, it is the best herb to allay your appetite. It will also reduce digestive disturbances such as dyspepsia, gas and flatulence.

Parsley, lemongrass and hibiscus are diuretic herbs that will help with fluid retention and cellulite.

Parsley is a powerful diuretic herb that is highly nutritive and calming to the stomach.

Lemongrass makes a refreshing and pleasant-tasting tea. It is helpful in the elimination of cellulite.

Hibiscus is often an ingredient in prepackaged teas along with **rose hip**. Both teas are a source of vitamin C, providing you make the tea with water that has not come to a boil, as vitamin C is destroyed at the boiling point.

Chamomile is a relaxing herb, and is very calming to a nervous stomach when combined with **peppermint**. Chamomile assists digestion by promoting bile and gastric secretions.

Nettle will help to stabilize blood sugar fluctuations and is highly nutritive. Drinking nettle tea will also relieve eczema and dermatitis.

Red bush tea is a very pleasant tea to drink. It is useful in allergic conditions and especially so for milk allergy. I have included it with your body type because many gynecoid women have had a high intake of dairy products.

Dandelion is a wonderful coffee substitute that is especially good for your liver and kidneys. If you have gallbladder or liver problems, this herb is for you. It is also useful if you have a high blood cholesterol level.

LYMPHATIC SHAPE—
HERBAL TEAS

Herbal teas suit your body type well. You need to avoid dairy products so cups of tea (containing tannin) and coffee are best avoided, especially if you are used to drinking them with milk and sugar. Soy milk doesn't go down terribly well in a cup of tannin tea.

There are several herbs that will work especially well for you.

Red bush tea is specific for milk allergy and, as you know by now, dairy products are not metabolized well in your body. A pleasant and refreshing tea to drink (very popular in Australia), it can be purchased in tea bags for convenience. It is a tonic and is useful for treating mild gastric complaints.

Lemongrass will be refreshing on a hot day and is a mild diuretic that helps with fluid retention and the elimination of cellulite.

Blue flag is an attractive lily with violet flowers. In some countries it is called "liver lily" because of its action on that organ. It will help to decongest your lymphatic system and promote the flow of bile, saliva and gastric secretions. Because of this it is wonderful for your sluggish metabolism and constipation.

Rose hip and hibiscus teas are often used in combination in prepackaged teas. They are refreshing and highly nutritive, and are both a good source of vitamin C, which naturally helps to mobilize fats.

Dandelion tea is made from the ground roots of this herb. It is a good coffee substitute that is a tonic to the liver and kidneys. It will help your body metabolize cholesterol and it will improve your digestion. It will improve chronic constipation and is also beneficial for rheumatism.

Nettle tea will help with fluctuations in blood sugar levels and can slightly lower blood pressure. It is highly nutritive and can heal itchy skin conditions such as nervous eczema and dermatitis.

Ginger is a stimulant herb that has a special affinity with digestion. It is great for flatulent dyspepsia or colic. You may wish to add a teaspoon of ginger powder to red bush tea and sip slowly.

Fennel tea is a slimming aid. It allays hunger and will be useful to drink during your danger times for snacks. Use the fresh or dried leaves and seeds to make the tea.

Parsley tea is calming to the stomach and helps to sweeten your breath. It is nutritive and is a powerful diuretic that assists elimination of edema or fluid retention.

THYROID SHAPE— HERBAL TEAS

The herbs I have chosen for your body shape are a selection that will stabilize blood sugar fluctuations and regulate your metabolic rate.

Valerian tea makes a relaxing drink that is very calming to your digestive system. It is beneficial to your nervous system and will help if you are experiencing anxiety or insomnia. It is useful for the treatment of migraine headaches or nervous exhaustion.

Chamomile is another tea that has a mild sedative action. It has a special affinity for the stomach and when it is made as a weak tea it acts as a tonic.

Licorice root is a great tea for you. It strengthens your burnt-out adrenals and provides you with a pleasant, sweet-tasting drink. It will help to regulate your blood sugar levels and keep your energy steady.

If you have made a decision to stop smoking, then licorice root tea will be very helpful in clearing the bronchial tubes and lungs of mucus, as it is a powerful expectorant.

Fenugreek tea is a good tonic and can stimulate your appetite. I see no danger in this as women with your body type often have little desire to eat regular meals and tend to make the wrong choices when their blood sugar levels drop too low. Fenugreek will help you to form better eating patterns.

Nettle also stabilizes blood sugar levels and is a nutritive tonic herb.

Rosemary is the herb of remembrance. It may improve your memory and is used specifically to treat migraine headaches. It can reduce blood pressure slightly and has a mild sedative action.

Fennel is included in case you get hungry at the wrong times. It will allay your hunger and calm your digestion.

Alfalfa is a great herb to alkalize an overacid stomach. It is highly nutritive and is a wonderful tonic.

Lemon balm is a tea that helps to treat nervous palpitations and restlessness. Thyroid fluctuations often lead to depressive states, and lemon balm will help to lift your spirits.

Passion flower is another sedative herb that has an action on the adrenals. This tea will help to relax you without leaving you tired.

PART THREE

BODY-SHAPING RECIPES

CHAPTER FIFTEEN

RECImPES

APPETIZERS

STUFFED MUSHROOM CAPS

Allow 3 mushrooms per person.
Remove the stems and wipe the caps with a damp cloth.
Place upside down in a shallow baking dish ready for filling.

SAUCE
2 teaspoons melted low-fat margarine
1 tablespoon whole wheat flour
1 cup low-fat 2% calcium-enriched or soy milk
½ bunch freshly cooked asparagus or drained 12-ounce can asparagus, cut into pieces
Paprika

Combine the margarine and flour in a small saucepan and stir over moderate heat for 1 minute. Add the milk and continue stirring until the mixture boils and thickens. Add the cooked asparagus pieces and blend. Fill or cover the mushrooms and sprinkle with paprika. Bake or grill until hot and bubbly.

APPROXIMATELY 65 CALORIES PER SERVING

EGG AND TUNA COMBO

2 hard-boiled eggs, chopped
8 ounces tuna in spring water, drained and mashed with a fork
½ cup low-fat cottage cheese
1 shallot, finely chopped
2 teaspoons chopped fresh dill
2 teaspoons chopped parsley
Cayenne pepper or paprika (optional)

Combine all the ingredients and serve with toasted whole grain bread, crackers or pita bread.

TOTAL CALORIES (EXCLUDING BREAD) ARE APPROXIMATELY 556. MAKES APPROXIMATELY 1⅔ CUPS OR 28 TABLESPOONS (1 SERVING = 1 TABLESPOON).

DEVILED EGGS

6 free-range eggs
2 teaspoons light mayonnaise
1 teaspoon Dijon mustard
1 teaspoon curry powder
Fresh mint and parsley, finely chopped, to garnish

Hard-boil the eggs, peel them and allow to cool. Cut the eggs in half lengthwise and remove the yolks. Mash the yolks with the mayonnaise, mustard and curry powder in a small bowl and place spoonfuls back into each egg half. Garnish with a little parsley and mint.

Serves 6 (APPROXIMATELY 80 CALORIES PER SERVING)

GUACAMOLE

This recipe can be used as a dip with unsalted crackers or fresh chopped raw vegetables. I suggest a platter that contains broccoli florets, carrot sticks, zucchini sticks, green pepper, celery, fennel and radish. A large plateful of these vegetables would yield 80 to 100 calories.

1 medium avocado
3 garlic cloves, finely chopped
Lemon or lime juice to taste

Mash the avocado and garlic together with a fork. Mix in some lemon or lime juice to flavor the dish. Guacamole mixture should have a smooth but firm consistency. You may add a little fresh chili to this recipe, if desired.

Serves 2 to 4 (TOTAL CALORIES APPROXIMATELY 325)

HUMMUS

This vegetarian dish is an excellent addition to a salad, can be eaten as a dip or an alternative spread on crackers or bread. It is a good source of protein, calcium and vitamin C.

10–11 ounces cooked chickpeas
⅓ cup tahini (sesame paste)
3 garlic cloves, chopped
Juice of 2 to 3 lemons
Freshly ground black pepper
Paprika (optional)

Blend or grind the chickpeas until smooth. Add all the other ingredients to the blender and combine thoroughly.

Add more tahini or lemon juice as necessary to suit your taste and to reach a smooth but not runny consistency. Place in a serving dish and sprinkle with paprika, if desired. Makes approximately 1¼ cups or 40 tablespoons.

1 TABLESPOON CONTAINS 60 CALORIES.

BABAGANOUJ

2 pounds eggplant
3 garlic cloves
Juice of 2 lemons
⅓ cup tahini (sesame paste)
Roasted sesame seeds to garnish

Bake in a moderate oven (350°F.) or grill whole eggplants (if grilling use small eggplants) until the skin blisters and turns black (30 minutes). Peel the eggplants while they are still hot.

Blend the eggplant pulp with the garlic, lemon juice and tahini. You may wish to taste the mixture and add more lemon juice or garlic to suit your palate. Place in a dish, sprinkle with roasted sesame seeds and chill.

Serve with pita bread, rice crackers or fresh raw vegetables.

Serves 6 to 8 (APPROXIMATELY 90 TO 120 CALORIES PER SERVING)

SOUPS

MINESTRONE SOUP

1 onion, chopped
2 potatoes, diced
3 garlic cloves
15 ounces canned peeled tomatoes, finely chopped or
    equivalent fresh
1 tablespoon chopped parsley
2 medium carrots, diced
1 celery stalk, thinly sliced
1½ cups beef stock
2 cups water
11 ounces canned cannellini beans

Place all the ingredients except the beans in a saucepan and bring to a boil. Reduce the heat and simmer for 30 to 45 minutes; add the beans and cook another 15 minutes.

Serves 6 to 8 (75 CALORIES PER SERVING)

ZUCCHINI SOUP

1½ pounds zucchini, sliced
2 celery stalks, thinly sliced
1 carrot, diced
1 potato, diced
1 onion, finely chopped
2 cups water
1 cup chicken stock
½ cup soy milk
1 tablespoon chopped parsley or 1 teaspoon dried
1 tablespoon chopped fresh basil or 1 teaspoon dried
Freshly ground black pepper

Bring all the ingredients except the soy milk, parsley, basil and pepper to a boil in a large saucepan. Reduce the heat and simmer until the vegetables are just cooked (20 to 25 minutes). Remove from the heat and blenderize with the soy milk. Add the parsley, basil and lots of black pepper. Do not boil when reheating.

Serves 6 (55 CALORIES PER SERVING)

SQUASH SOUP

1 butternut squash, peeled and cut into pieces
1 onion, chopped
1 potato, diced
1 celery stalk, thinly sliced
3 garlic cloves, minced
½ teaspoon nutmeg
1 tablespoon chopped fresh coriander or 1 teaspoon dried

1½ cups water
1 cup chicken stock
½ cup soy milk
Plain low-fat yogurt and fresh parsley to garnish

Bring all the ingredients except the soy milk, yogurt and parsley to a boil, then reduce the heat and simmer until the vegetables are cooked. Blenderize with the soy milk and serve with a dollop of yogurt and fresh parsley.

Serves 6 to 8 (100 CALORIES PER SERVING)

ITALIAN NOODLE SOUP

6½ cups water
2 small onions
1 handful of Italian parsley
Coriander sprigs
1 handful of fresh basil
2 large potatoes
2 carrots
2 celery stalks
1 parsnip
1 turnip
1 bay leaf
Small handful of chives
Freshly ground black pepper
½ cup red lentils
½ cup brown lentils
11-ounce can cannellini beans
26-ounce can V8 vegetable juice
1 garlic clove

1 tablespoon tomato paste
1 pound canned tomatoes or equivalent fresh
1 tablespoon vegetable bouillon, mixed to a paste with
   some hot water
1 tablespoon low-sodium soy sauce
1⅔ cups chicken stock
½ cup soup noodles (small pasta)

Prepare a stock with the water, 1 onion and all the vegetable skins and tops. Boil for about half an hour and strain, reserving the liquid.

Blend the onions, parsley, coriander and basil into a paste, then combine with the stock in a large pot.

Chop the remaining vegetables and herbs very finely and add to the stock. Add the pepper, lentils, beans, V8 juice, garlic, tomato paste, tomatoes, vegetable stock, soy sauce and chicken stock. Cover and cook over low heat for 1 hour. Stir the pot occasionally. Add the noodles and cook for an additional half hour.

Serves 8 (175 CALORIES PER SERVING)

SALADS

TABBOULI SALAD

1 cup bulgur or cracked wheat
3 shallots, chopped
1 bunch of parsley, about 4 ounces, finely chopped
½ cup finely chopped fresh mint
Juice of 2 lemons
3 tomatoes, diced

Place the bulgur in a bowl and cover with cold water. Leave to soak for 30 minutes. Drain, press out excess water and leave to dry for 30 minutes.

Place the bulgur in a bowl and combine with the other ingredients. Lightly toss and serve immediately.

Serves 4 (APPROXIMATELY 120 CALORIES PER SERVING)

FRESH ASPARAGUS VINAIGRETTE

12 fresh asparagus spears

DRESSING
1 tablespoon pine nuts
2 shallots, finely chopped
2 teaspoons finely chopped fresh tarragon or parsley
1 garlic clove, finely chopped
1 tablespoon cold-pressed olive oil
1 tablespoon white wine vinegar or lime juice
1 teaspoon honey

Trim the thick, coarse ends from the asparagus. Lightly steam, taking care not to overcook. Rinse quickly under cold water to retain color and arrange on a serving platter.

Lightly roast the pine nuts in a microwave or skillet and set aside. Combine all the other ingredients in a glass container and whisk lightly. Pour over the asparagus and scatter the pine nuts on top.

Serves 4 (APPROXIMATELY 75 CALORIES PER SERVING)

GREEN VEGETABLE PLATE

Arrange a combination of raw and steamed green vegetables on a platter or large dinner plate. A good combination would be:

4 fresh asparagus spears
8 snow peas
8 whole green beans
4 broccoli florets
4 button squash
½ small avocado, sliced
Raw zucchini sticks

Serves 4 to 6 (APPROXIMATELY 70 CALORIES PER SERVING)

DUKKAH

Our Mustard Vinaigrette (page 188) may be served with this dish.

In a heavy skillet, roast ½ cup of mixed coarsely chopped pine nuts, cashews, hazelnuts or macadamia nuts, sesame and sunflower seeds. Add 1 teaspoon lightly crushed, roasted coriander seeds and mix together. The combined quantity yields ½ cup. Place in a small bowl and serve with vegetables.

Serves 4 (APPROXIMATELY 125 CALORIES PER SERVING)

MIXED BEAN AND RICE SALAD

½ cup canned four-bean mix
1 cup cold cooked brown rice
1 medium onion, finely chopped
3 shallots, finely chopped
½ red pepper, diced
½ cup corn kernels
1 handful of parsley, finely chopped
A few sun-dried tomatoes, finely sliced
¼ cup raisins
¼ cup Hazelnut Dressing (page 190)

Combine all the salad ingredients in a serving bowl, add the dressing and toss well.

Serves 2 (APPROXIMATELY 400 CALORIES PER SERVING)

PASTA SALAD

2 cups cooked macaroni
1 celery stalk, finely chopped
8 cherry tomatoes, halved
2 tablespoons chopped parsley
2 shallots, finely chopped
½ red pepper, thinly sliced
3 radishes, sliced
⅓ cup sliced mushrooms
2 small sliced zucchini
5 tablespoons Vinaigrette Dressing (page 189)

Combine all the salad ingredients in a serving bowl, add the dressing and toss well.

Serves 4 (APPROXIMATELY 170 CALORIES PER SERVING)

BEET AND WATERCRESS SALAD

2 medium beets
2 large red onions
Lettuce leaves
1 bunch watercress or arugula
6 radishes

Cook and slice fresh beets, leave to cool, or use 1½ cups drained sliced canned beets.

Thinly slice the onions and place in a bowl. Pour over some boiling water and let stand for 1 minute, then drain.

Arrange the lettuce leaves in a bowl or on a plate. Top with the beets, onion, watercress and sliced radishes. Sprinkle with the dressing of your choice or fresh lemon juice.

Serves 8 (APPROXIMATELY 20 CALORIES PER SERVING)

GREEN BEAN AND APPLE SALAD

1 large Granny Smith apple
¼ cup No Oil Dressing (page 189)
1 pound green beans, ends snapped off
1 red onion, thinly sliced
1 red pepper, sliced or chopped
1 tablespoon finely chopped parsley

1 tablespoon finely chopped fresh mint or 1 teaspoon
  dried
6 lettuce leaves
1 cup alfalfa sprouts

Core the apple, dice into bite-sized cubes and place in a
small bowl. Pour over No Oil Dressing. Marinate while you
wash and prepare the other ingredients.

Place all the ingredients in a large bowl and toss lightly.

Serves 8 (APPROXIMATELY 60 CALORIES PER SERVING)

CARROT AND RAISIN SALAD

3 large carrots, grated
¼ green pepper, chopped
⅓ cup seedless raisins
1 tablespoon sunflower seeds.
2 tablespoons Sweet Walnut Dressing, made with orange
  juice (page 191)

Combine all the salad ingredients and toss well with the
dressing.

Serves 6 (APPROXIMATELY 90 CALORIES PER SERVING)

SPINACH AND WALNUT SALAD

Some raisins are a nice addition to this salad.

6 spinach leaves, stems removed
Nutmeg (optional)

3 shallots, finely chopped
¼ cup Sweet Walnut Dressing (page 191)

Lightly steam the spinach for 2 minutes, chop coarsely and set aside to cool. Sprinkle with a little nutmeg, if desired. Lightly toss the shallots and dressing through the spinach.

Serves 6 (APPROXIMATELY 60 CALORIES PER SERVING)

SLIMMERS' EGG AND POTATO SALAD

3 large potatoes, scrubbed, diced and cooked
1 onion, finely chopped
4 hard-boiled eggs, sliced
1 tablespoon finely chopped parsley
1 tablespoon finely chopped mint or 1 teaspoon dried
1 cup plain low-fat yogurt
Sprinkle of cayenne pepper
Green pepper rings to garnish

Combine all the salad ingredients in a large bowl and lightly toss. Garnish with green pepper rings.

Serves 6 (APPROXIMATELY 175 CALORIES PER SERVING)

GREEK SALAD

2 cups shredded lettuce
1 tomato, thinly sliced
1 small cucumber, sliced
½ green pepper, sliced

1 onion, thinly sliced
4 ounces feta cheese, cut into small cubes
8 black olives
½ cup No Oil Dressing (page 189)
Finely chopped fresh mint to garnish
Finely chopped parsley to garnish
Finely chopped fresh basil to garnish

Arrange a bed of lettuce on a large plate. Place a layer of sliced tomatoes on top, followed by sliced cucumber, green pepper and onion. Top with feta cheese and olives. Pour the dressing over and sprinkle with fresh herbs.

Serves 2 (APPROXIMATELY 265 CALORIES PER SERVING)

MUSHROOM AND SNOW PEA SALAD

4.5 ounces mushrooms
12 snow peas
2 spring onions, sliced
Juice of 1 lemon or lime
2 teaspoons olive oil
8 roasted hazelnuts, roughly chopped

Wipe the mushrooms, trim the stems and slice thinly. Place in a bowl with the washed, whole snow peas and spring onions. Combine the lemon juice and oil and pour over the salad vegetables. Sprinkle with hazelnuts and lightly toss the salad.

Serves 2 (APPROXIMATELY 100 CALORIES PER SERVING)

MARINATED SCALLOPS

1 pound sea scallops

MARINADE
¼ cup soy sauce
2 tablespoons light olive oil
2 tablespoons honey
1 tablespoon vinegar
Pinch of ground ginger
1 to 2 garlic cloves, crushed

Wash the scallops and pat them dry. Bring a saucepan of water to a boil and quickly cook the scallops (4 to 6 minutes). Do not overcook. Drain the scallops and set aside.

Combine all the marinade ingredients in a large bowl and add the cooked scallops. Marinate for 15 minutes. Serve on a bed of hot rice.

Serves 4 (200 CALORIES PER SERVING; 365 CALORIES PER SERVING WITH ¾ CUP RICE)

SEAFOOD SALAD

4 ounces cooked fish or shellfish (canned or fresh), roughly chopped
2 shallots, finely chopped
½-inch piece gingerroot, finely chopped
1 red chili, seeded and finely chopped
8 roasted cashew nuts, roughly chopped
1 mango, roughly chopped
¼ cup Tangy Lime Dressing (page 188)

Lettuce leaves
Cherry tomatoes and mint leaves to garnish
Rice (optional)

Combine all the ingredients together in a medium bowl with the dressing. Serve immediately on washed lettuce leaves. Garnish with cherry tomatoes and mint leaves. Serve with rice, if desired.

Serves 2 (260 CALORIES PER SERVING; 425 CALORIES PER SERVING WITH ¾ CUP RICE)

LIME CHICKEN SALAD

2 chicken breasts, grilled and cut into small cubes
2 shallots, finely chopped
½ green pepper, finely chopped
2 red chilies, seeded and finely chopped
¼ cup Sweet Lime Dressing (page 189)
Lettuce leaves
1 tablespoon chopped mint
Freshly ground black pepper
Rice (optional)

Combine the chicken, shallots, green pepper and chilies in a medium bowl. Toss with the dressing, then serve on washed lettuce leaves and garnish with mint. Sprinkle with pepper. Serve with rice, if desired.

Serves 4 (155 CALORIES PER SERVING; 335 CALORIES PER SERVING WITH ¾ CUP RICE)

FRUIT AND CHICKEN SALAD

2 chicken breasts, grilled and cut into small cubes
2 tablespoons roughly chopped almonds
1 cup seedless white grapes
2 red chilies, seeded and finely chopped
3 shallots, chopped
1 tablespoon chopped fresh mint or coriander
½ cup Ginger Dressing (page 188)

Combine all the ingredients in a bowl and lightly toss with the dressing. Serve with steamed or boiled rice.

Serves 4 (190 CALORIES PER SERVING; 355 CALORIES PER SERVING WITH ¾ CUP RICE)

CUCUMBER SALAD

Cucumbers are rich in vitamin A, potassium, calcium and phosphorus. This dish from Thailand turns a simple vegetable into a very tasty, refreshing salad.

2 medium cucumbers
2 teaspoons sugar
2 tablespoons white vinegar
1 red chili, seeded and finely chopped
1 heaping tablespoon roughly chopped almonds or pecan nuts
2 shallots, finely chopped
1 tablespoon chopped fresh coriander

Wash the cucumbers and slice horizontally through the middle. Leave the skin on and carefully scoop out the seeds. Finely slice the cucumbers and place in a serving bowl.

Combine the sugar and vinegar and stir until the sugar has dissolved. Pour over the cucumber and mix well.

Sprinkle the chili, nuts, shallots and coriander on top and allow to marinate for 1 hour.

Serves 4 (APPROXIMATELY 60 CALORIES PER SERVING)

DRESSINGS

The general rule when preparing a dressing is to start with the vinegar or juice and add the seasoning. Whisk together and slowly add the oil, a little at a time, beating as you go. Nuts and fresh herbs should be added last.

A dash of water added to your salad dressing will make it go further and reduce the pungency of the vinegar.

I have significantly reduced the amount of oil that is usually used in recipes for salad dressing to reduce calories.

I encourage you to be creative and experiment with different types of vinegars, juices, herbs, seasonings and nuts to alter the flavor and sharpness of your dressing.

Fruit vinegars are delicious on salads that contain fruit.

You may simply wish to squeeze a little fresh lemon or lime juice over your salad. This will increase your vitamin C levels and add a few extra enzymes to aid digestion.

SPICY THAI DRESSING

2 stalks lemongrass, chopped
3 chilies, seeded, if desired, and chopped

¼ cup lime or lemon juice
1 tablespoon fish sauce*

30 CALORIES/APPROXIMATELY ⅓ CUP

TANGY LIME DRESSING

2 tablespoons lime juice
1 tablespoon lime zest
2 tablespoons fish sauce*

40 CALORIES/APPROXIMATELY ¼ CUP

GINGER DRESSING

⅓ cup lime juice
1 tablespoon fish sauce*
1 teaspoon brown sugar
1 teaspoon ground ginger

40 CALORIES/APPROXIMATELY ⅓ CUP

MUSTARD VINAIGRETTE

2 teaspoons light oil
Juice of 1 lime or lemon
1 teaspoon Dijon mustard
1 garlic clove, minced

100 CALORIES/APPROXIMATELY ⅓ CUP

SWEET LIME DRESSING

1 tablespoon fish sauce*
2 teaspoons sugar
2 tablespoons lime juice

50 CALORIES/APPROXIMATELY ¼ CUP

NO OIL DRESSING

½ cup red wine vinegar
Juice of 1 lemon or lime
2 garlic cloves, minced
Chopped chives
Freshly ground black pepper

40 CALORIES PER ¾ CUP
3 CALORIES PER TABLESPOON

VINAIGRETTE DRESSING

1 tablespoon light olive oil
1 tablespoon white wine vinegar or lemon juice
1 garlic clove, minced
Freshly ground black pepper

125 CALORIES PER APPROXIMATELY ⅛ CUP
42 CALORIES PER TABLESPOON

*Five-ounce bottles of fish sauce can be found in most supermarkets in the international, ethnic or Oriental food sections.

MOCK SOUR CREAM DRESSING

½ cup part-skim ricotta cheese
¼ cup plain low-fat yogurt
Chopped chives
Parsley and mint, if desired

200 CALORIES PER ¾ CUP
17 CALORIES PER TABLESPOON

HAZELNUT DRESSING

1 tablespoon light olive oil
1 tablespoon balsamic vinegar
2 teaspoons water
2 tablespoons coarsely chopped roasted hazelnuts
½ teaspoon ground ginger
½ teaspoon honey

200 CALORIES PER APPROXIMATELY ¼ CUP
43 CALORIES PER TABLESPOON

CORIANDER MAYONNAISE

½ cup plain low-fat yogurt
⅓ cup light mayonnaise
Chopped coriander
2 teaspoons Dijon mustard
2 teaspoons lemon juice
Freshly ground black pepper

300 CALORIES PER APPROXIMATELY 1 CUP
20 CALORIES PER TABLESPOON

RASPBERRY VINAIGRETTE

2 teaspoons raspberry vinegar
1 teaspoon lime juice
½ teaspoon Dijon mustard
1 tablespoon olive oil
2 tablespoons coarsely chopped pecan nuts

225 CALORIES PER ¼ CUP
55 CALORIES PER TABLESPOON

SWEET WALNUT DRESSING

1 tablespoon light olive oil
1 tablespoon lemon, lime, grapefruit or orange juice
2 tablespoons coarsely chopped walnuts
½ teaspoon honey
2 garlic cloves, minced

225 CALORIES PER APPROXIMATELY ¼ CUP
45 CALORIES PER TABLESPOON

SAUCES

EASY ONION SAUCE

Great to serve with chicken, fish or vegetables.

3 cups chopped onion
1 tablespoon skim milk or soy milk

½ teaspoon nutmeg
Freshly ground black pepper to taste
Lemon juice

Microwave or steam the onion and blend with the milk, nutmeg, black pepper and a dash of lemon juice.

Serves 4 (45 CALORIES PER SERVING)

CHILI SAUCE

1 chopped tomato
1 spring onion, finely chopped
1 seeded and chopped fresh chili or ½ teaspoon dried
2 teaspoons finely chopped parsley
2 teaspoons finely chopped coriander

Combine all the ingredients and cook until tender in a microwave. Or cook in a saucepan, stirring constantly over moderate heat.

Serves 1 (45 CALORIES)

BLENDER HOLLANDAISE

1 tablespoon light margarine, melted
1 egg yolk (raw)
Juice of 1 or 2 limes or lemons

Blend all the ingredients. Use immediately; it will not keep.

Serves 3 (APPROXIMATELY 50 CALORIES PER SERVING)

PARSLEY SAUCE

2 teaspoons light margarine
1 tablespoon whole wheat flour
1¼ cups low-fat 2% calcium-enriched milk
1 tablespoon finely chopped parsley
Freshly ground black pepper
A squeeze of lemon juice and 1 teaspoon grated lemon rind
Finely chopped onion or shallots (optional)

Melt the margarine in a small saucepan. Add the flour away from the heat and stir with a wooden spoon until smooth. Stir over low heat for 1 minute; it must not burn. Add the milk gradually, stirring well until the sauce boils and thickens. Add the parsley, pepper, lemon juice, lemon rind and finely chopped onion or shallots, if desired.

Serves 6 (APPROXIMATELY 40 CALORIES PER SERVING)

PESTO SAUCE

½ bunch fresh basil
1 tablespoon pine nuts
2 garlic cloves
2 teaspoons olive oil
Freshly ground black pepper

Blenderize all the ingredients and serve on cooked pasta or baked potatoes.

Serves 2 (APPROXIMATELY 115 CALORIES PER SERVING)

BASIC FOUNDATION SAUCE

This basic recipe is useful as a base for any sauce. Add less milk to make a thicker binding sauce for pies or fritters.

2 tablespoons low-fat margarine
2 tablespoons flour
1½ cups low-fat 2% calcium-enriched milk or soy milk
(or a combination for a creamier low-fat sauce that
does not have a strong soy taste)

Melt the margarine over low heat and stir in the flour. Cook for 2 minutes over low heat, stirring continuously. Add the milk gradually and stir until the sauce boils and thickens.

Serves 4 (APPROXIMATELY 90 CALORIES PER SERVING). TOTAL CALORIES FOR SAUCE ARE APPROXIMATELY 350.

VARIATIONS FOR BASIC FOUNDATION SAUCE

Many herbs can be added to change the sauce according to the food it is to accompany. Listed below are a few simple sauce ideas.

Mustard Sauce—Add 1 tablespoon prepared mustard to the sauce. Serve with corned beef or fish. Total: 400 calories.

Egg Sauce—Add 2 chopped hard-boiled eggs to the sauce. Serve with fish, chicken or corned beef. Total: 500 calories.

Mushroom Sauce—Cook ½ cup mushrooms and a little garlic in the microwave and add to the sauce. Total: 365 calories.

Florentine Sauce—Add a dash of Tabasco, Worcestershire sauce, nutmeg, parsley and 1 cup cooked, pureed spinach. Serve with fish, eggs, chicken or potato. Total: 400 calories.

Mornay Sauce—Add 2 tablespoons Parmesan cheese and a pat of margarine to the sauce as it thickens. Serve with fish, seafood, eggs and vegetables. Total: 670 calories.

Onion Sauce—Steam or microwave 2 finely chopped onions until tender and stir into the sauce. Good with beef or fish. Total: 400 calories.

TOMATO SALSA

2 tomatoes, diced
¼ green pepper, diced
1 small onion, finely chopped
3 or 4 fresh basil leaves, finely chopped
Chopped fresh parsley
½ fresh chili with seeds removed, finely chopped

Combine all the ingredients in a small bowl.

Serves 2 (APPROXIMATELY 45 CALORIES PER SERVING)

MINTED TOMATO SALSA

2 tomatoes, diced
1 small onion, finely chopped
2 teaspoons finely chopped fresh mint
2 teaspoons finely chopped parsley

Combine all the ingredients in a small bowl.

Serves 2 (APPROXIMATELY 35 CALORIES PER SERVING)

ENTRÉES

TANDOORI FISH

1 medium onion
6 garlic cloves
¾-inch piece fresh gingerroot
1 chili
Juice of 1 lemon
1 tablespoon ground coriander
1 teaspoon cumin
2 teaspoons fennel seeds
5 cardamom pods
1 teaspoon ground cinnamon
Freshly ground black pepper
1 teaspoon paprika
1 cup plain low-fat yogurt
1 whole fish, about 2 pounds
Lime slices to garnish
Fresh coriander to garnish

Blenderize the onion, garlic, ginger and chili until smooth.

Combine all the other spices and herbs* in a mortar and grind together. Add the spices and yogurt to the onion mixture and blend to a paste.

Make several diagonal incisions across the fish and rub on the paste, inside and out, to coat the fish. Refrigerate for 2 hours.

Grill, barbecue or bake the fish until the skin is crisp and

*Commercial tandoori mixture is available in some supermarkets and health food stores.

the flesh begins to flake, about 20 minutes depending on the size of the fish.

Garnish with lime slices and fresh coriander.

Serves 2 to 4 (APPROXIMATELY 300 TO 600 CALORIES PER SERVING)

CREAMY FISH ROLLS WITH DILL SAUCE

The enzymes in the fruit and fresh ginger in this recipe assist your digestion. If you dislike combining fruit with fish, then try using carrot and zucchini sticks or oysters as a filling instead.

8 thin white fish fillets
1 tablespoon finely chopped parsley and ½-inch piece finely chopped fresh gingerroot mixed into the juice of 1 lime or lemon
8 slices of fresh mango or cantaloupe
1 cup low-fat 2% calcium-enriched milk
2 teaspoons cornstarch
1 tablespoon chopped fresh dill

Brush 1 side of each fish fillet with the lime juice mixture. Roll each fillet (brushed side to middle) around a slice of fruit and secure with a toothpick or skewer. Place in a single layer in a shallow ovenproof dish. Pour over the milk, cover and poach in the microwave for about 8 minutes, or in a moderate oven (425°F.) for 15 to 20 minutes, until the fish is just cooked. DO NOT OVERCOOK. Carefully remove the fish rolls with a slotted spoon and set aside in a warm place while the sauce is made from pan juices.

Blend the cornstarch with a little cold low-fat calcium-enriched milk to make a smooth paste. Strain the pan juices and place in a small saucepan. Add the blended cornstarch and stir constantly over moderate heat until the mixture boils and thickens. Add the chopped fresh dill and serve immediately over the fish rolls.

Serves 8 (APPROXIMATELY 125 CALORIES PER SERVING)

BAKED STUFFED FISH

1 cup cooked brown rice
2 shallots, chopped
⅓ cup chopped celery
1 teaspoon paprika
½-inch piece fresh gingerroot
2 to 3 pounds whole fish such as snapper, rainbow trout or perch
Lemon or lime juice
Fennel tips, lemon or lime slices and some fresh ginger cut into thin slices to garnish

In a small bowl, combine the cooked rice, shallots, celery, paprika and ginger. Stuff the cleaned and scaled fish with this mixture and place in a baking dish. Squeeze over fresh lemon or lime juice and garnish with fennel, citrus slices and ginger. Pour ¼ cup water into the dish and cover with foil or a lid to stop the fish from drying out. Bake in a moderate oven (350°F.) until the fish is just cooked, approximately 35 minutes.

Serves 5 (APPROXIMATELY 250 CALORIES PER SERVING)

PORK AND PINEAPPLE KEBABS

3 ounces pork fillet
2 slices fresh pineapple
1 onion
½ cup fresh mushrooms
6 cherry tomatoes

Cut all the ingredients except the tomatoes into bite-sized pieces and thread alternately onto bamboo or metal skewers. Grill or barbecue until the meat is cooked to your liking.

Serves 1 (APPROXIMATELY 315 CALORIES)

LAMB AND FRUIT KEBABS

3.5 ounces lamb steak
3 apricots or 1 small mango
1 onion
6 fresh mushrooms
6 cherry tomatoes

Cut all the ingredients exccpt the tomatoes into bite-sized pieces and thread alternately onto bamboo or metal skewers. Grill or barbecue until the meat is cooked to your liking.

Serves 1 (APPROXIMATELY 400 CALORIES)

MARINATED CHICKEN KEBABS

MARINADE:
1 onion
¼ cup white cooking wine
2 tablespoons vinegar
1 tablespoon dried rosemary or marjoram
2 garlic cloves
3 skinless chicken breasts

Combine all marinade ingredients.

Trim all fat from the chicken and cut into bite-sized pieces. Place the meat in the marinade and coat each piece of chicken thoroughly. Marinate for 1 hour.

Thread the chicken onto bamboo or metal skewers and grill or barbecue until cooked (5 to 8 minutes).

Serves 6 (145 CALORIES PER SERVING)

BRAISED STEAK

12 ounces skirt steak or stew beef
3 celery stalks
2 large carrots
2 medium onions
Mixed herbs
1½ cups beef stock
½ cup water

Cut the steak into 8 equal portions and slice the vegetables into large pieces. Heat a little water in a large casserole dish over moderate heat. Quickly brown the meat in the water to seal in the juices and set aside.

Place the vegetables, herbs, stock and the water into the casserole dish. Stir to combine and place the meat carefully on top in order to cook it above the vegetables. Seal with a tight-fitting lid and bring to a boil.

Reduce the heat and simmer with the lid on for 2 hours.

Serves 4 (APPROXIMATELY 290 CALORIES PER SERVING)

IRISH STEW

12 small potatoes
3 carrots
1 teaspoon vegetable bouillon
½ cup warm water
4 sprigs of fresh oregano
1 bunch of finely chopped parsley
3 onions
2½ pounds lamb steaks or fillets
4 tomatoes or 1 8-ounce can tomatoes
1 tablespoon low-sodium soy sauce
Freshly ground black pepper
2 celery stalks, finely chopped

Scrub the potatoes and carrots. Cut the potatoes in half and line the bottom of a large casserole dish or saucepan with them. Dissolve the vegetable bouillon in the warm water and pour over. Sprinkle with a handful of herbs and arrange a layer of the finely sliced onion rings. Place the meat on top, then the tomatoes, followed by the soy sauce, pepper and the remaining vegetables and herbs. Cover with a tight-fitting lid and cook over low heat for 1½ to 2 hours. Give the pot a light stir every 15 minutes to prevent burning.

Serves 8 (APPROXIMATELY 375 CALORIES PER SERVING)

CHICKEN AND VEGETABLE HOT POT

3¾ cups tomato or V8 vegetable juice
12 potatoes, scrubbed and halved
½ bunch of fresh basil, finely chopped
1 handful of parsley, finely chopped
Freshly ground black pepper
2 celery stalks, thinly sliced
2 large onions, sliced
8 chicken thigh fillets, trimmed of fat
32 ounces canned tomatoes or equivalent fresh, chopped
3 carrots, chopped
2 zucchini, chopped
1 parsnip, chopped
12 ounces squash, chopped
2 bay leaves
2 tablespoons low-sodium soy sauce
1 large teaspoon vegetable bouillon dissolved in ½ cup water
½ pound green beans, snapped

Pour a little V8 vegetable juice into the bottom of a heavy saucepan. Arrange the potatoes over the bottom of the pot and sprinkle with some of the basil, parsley and black pepper. Next arrange some celery and onion rings over the herbs, followed by the chicken fillets. Pour over half the chopped tomatoes. Arrange the carrots, zucchini, parsnip and squash in layers, with the onions on top, sprinkling each layer with the remaining basil, parsley and black pepper. Pour over the remaining tomatoes and add the bay leaves, soy sauce and dissolved vegetable bouillon. Lastly place the green beans on top. Check the level of juice in the pot; it should be one inch below the highest layer of the vegetables (add more V8 juice if needed).

Cover and cook over low heat, for 1½ to 2 hours. At 15-minute intervals shake the pot, lid on and all. It is an old Italian custom—and prevents burning.

Serves 8 (APPROXIMATELY 350 CALORIES PER SERVING)

CHICKEN AND MUSHROOM PIE

PIECRUST
1½ cups cooked brown rice
2 teaspoons oil
1 tablespoon chopped parsley
1 tablespoon sesame seeds (optional)

SAUCE
2 teaspoons low-fat margarine
1 tablespoon flour
Freshly ground black pepper
1 clove garlic, minced
¼ cup low-fat 2% calcium-enriched milk or soy milk
¼ cup chicken stock

FILLING
1 pound cooked chicken, cut into bite-sized pieces, with skin, bones and any visible fat removed
2 tablespoons thinly sliced red pepper

½ cup chopped broccoli florets
4 shallots, finely chopped
4 ounces fresh mushrooms
2 tablespoons chopped parsley
2 teaspoons chopped fresh rosemary or basil or 1 teaspoon dried
Any leftover cooked vegetables

TOPPING
1 cup cooked, mashed sweet potato
Sesame seeds (optional)

Combine all the piecrust ingredients and press the mixture into an ungreased pie dish.

To prepare the sauce, melt the margarine over low heat. Add the flour, pepper and garlic away from the heat and stir until combined well with the margarine. Return to the heat and stir over low heat for 1 minute. Add the milk and stock and stir continuously until the sauce boils and thickens.

In a large bowl, combine all the filling ingredients (plus extra vegetables if desired) and stir in the prepared sauce. Fill the piecrust with the mixture, top with the mashed sweet potato and sprinkle with sesame seeds, if desired. Bake in a moderate oven (350°F.) for 30 to 40 minutes.

Serves 6 (330 CALORIES PER SERVING)

AVOCADO AND CHICKEN IN FILO

2 chicken breasts, cut in half
8 sheets filo pastry
⅓ cup plain low-fat yogurt
1 small avocado, sliced

Lemon juice
Freshly ground black pepper
Tarragon, basil or marjoram
2 tablespoons low-fat margarine
1 tablespoon sesame seeds

Lightly pound the chicken breasts to an even thickness. Brush one sheet of filo with a little yogurt and cover with a second sheet. Brush again and fold in half to form a square. Place a piece of chicken diagonally at a corner of the pastry and top with avocado slices, lemon juice, pepper and your choice of herbs. Fold in half, roll up into a pastry parcel, tucking the ends under as you go. Repeat with the remaining chicken and filo. Place on a lightly greased baking tray and brush with a little melted low-fat margarine. Sprinkle with sesame seeds and bake in a moderate oven (350°F.) for 20 to 25 minutes, or until the pastry is golden brown.

Serves 4 (APPROXIMATELY 350 CALORIES PER SERVING)

CABBAGE ROLLS

¼ cup dark buckwheat
8 cabbage leaves
1 cup cooked chickpeas
½ cup plain low-fat yogurt
1 cup cooked brown rice
½ cup chopped fresh mushrooms
½ cup chopped celery
2 shallots, finely chopped
1 tablespoon chopped parsley
1 tablespoon chopped mint or 1 teaspoon dried

1 tablespoon chopped fresh marjoram or chopped basil
   or 1 teaspoon dried

SAUCE
3 large ripe tomatoes or 1 pound canned peeled tomatoes
1 onion, finely chopped
1 tablespoon chopped fresh basil or marjoram

Soak the buckwheat in warm water for 30 minutes to soften.
Strain and set aside. Trim thick stalks from the cabbage
leaves and steam until just tender. Do not overcook.

Puree the chickpeas in a blender with the yogurt. In a large
bowl, combine the chickpea puree, brown rice, buckwheat,
mushrooms, celery, shallots and herbs. Divide the mixture
into 8 portions and place each portion onto a precooked
cabbage leaf. Fold and roll up the mixture into each leaf,
tucking in the ends as you go to form small parcels. Place
in a single layer in a casserole dish.

To prepare the sauce, puree the tomatoes in a blender and
add the onion and basil or marjoram. Pour the sauce over
the rolls, cover and bake in a moderate oven (350°F.) for
30 minutes.

Serves 4 (APPROXIMATELY 225 CALORIES PER SERVING)

KIDNEY BEAN BAKE

9 ounces canned red kidney beans, drained
1 carrot, grated
1 celery stalk, finely chopped
1 cup part-skim ricotta cheese
1 tablespoon finely chopped parsley
2 teaspoons finely chopped fresh basil

Freshly ground black pepper
2 onions, finely sliced
⅔ cup vegetable stock
1 cup cooked, mashed sweet potato
Roasted sesame seeds (optional)

To the drained beans, mix in the grated carrot and celery. Lightly mix the ricotta cheese, parsley, basil and black pepper together.

Steam the onions until soft.

Put a third of the bean mixture into a greased ovenproof dish. Top with half the sliced onions and half the ricotta cheese. Repeat with another layer of beans and the remaining onion and ricotta. Finish with a layer of beans. Pour over the vegetable stock. Top with the mashed sweet potato and sprinkle over the sesame seeds, if desired. Bake in a moderate oven (350°F.) for 30 minutes.

Serves 4 (APPROXIMATELY 260 CALORIES PER SERVING)

OVEN-BAKED FALAFEL

Traditionally from the Middle East, falafels are delicious served with flat bread, Hummus (page 171) and Tabbouli Salad (page 176). This combination of foods provides a good source of protein and calcium.

Falafels are usually deep-fried, so take care with calories if you have not made them yourself.

¼ cup dark buckwheat
7 ounces cooked chickpeas
1 onion, finely chopped
2 shallots, finely chopped

3 garlic cloves, minced
1 tablespoon chopped parsley
2 teaspoons chopped mint
Fresh coriander (optional)
Freshly ground black pepper
¼ cup whole wheat flour
1 egg
1 tablespoon lemon juice
¼ cup sesame seeds

Soak the buckwheat in hot water for 10 minutes and drain well.

Finely grind or blend the chickpeas and add all the other ingredients, except the sesame seeds, and mix thoroughly. Cover and chill for 1 hour.

With wet hands, shape the mixture into individual patties and roll them in sesame seeds. Let sit 10 minutes more and bake in a moderate oven (350°F.) until golden brown, approximately 15–20 minutes, turning once.

Serves 6 (APPROXIMATELY 55 CALORIES PER SERVING)

LENTIL PATTIES

It is possible to substitute other beans in this recipe without affecting the calories.

1 pound cooked lentils, drained and mashed or coarsely
   blended with 1 tablespoon tahini (sesame paste)
½ cup cooked brown rice
1 celery stalk, finely chopped
1 carrot, grated
1 onion, finely chopped

3 garlic cloves, minced
1 tablespoon chopped parsley
1 tablespoon chopped fresh coriander or 1 teaspoon dried
Freshly ground black pepper
1 egg
Sesame seeds

Mix together all the ingredients except the sesame seeds.
Add some whole wheat flour if the mixture is too sloppy.
Form into patties and roll in the sesame seeds. Refrigerate
for 15 minutes so patties hold together better when cooking.
Cook in a nonstick pan with a smear of olive oil until golden
brown, turning once.

MAKES 10 TO 12 PATTIES (APPROXIMATELY 100 CALORIES PER
PATTY)

QUICK MEXICAN BEANS

15 ounces canned red kidney beans, drained
15 ounces peeled tomatoes, roughly chopped
½ green pepper, diced
1 onion, chopped
1 carrot, grated
1 celery stalk, finely chopped
¾ cup water
2 teaspoons chopped fresh basil or ¾ teaspoon dried

Place all of the ingredients in a saucepan and cook until
tender and thick (approximately 30 minutes), stirring occasionally.

Serves 6 (APPROXIMATELY 100 CALORIES PER SERVING)

DAHL

Any vegetables can be used in this dish. Dahl is a good source of protein when combined with brown rice.

3 cups water
½ pound red lentils
1 potato, diced
3.5 ounces sweet potato, diced
3.5 ounces squash, diced
1 onion, finely chopped
1 tablespoon curry powder or paste
1 tablespoon low-sodium soy sauce

Heat the water until boiling, then add the lentils, vegetables, curry and soy sauce. Reduce the heat and cook until the vegetables are soft and the dahl has thickened (about 20 to 30 minutes), stirring occasionally. Blend until smooth and serve.

Serves 2 to 4 (APPROXIMATELY 125 TO 250 CALORIES PER SERVING; 500 CALORIES TOTAL)

BUTTERNUT AND CASHEW QUICHE

PIECRUST
1½ cups cooked brown rice
1 tablespoon chopped parsley
2 teaspoons olive oil
1 tablespoon sesame seeds

FILLING
6 eggs
½ cup low-fat 2% calcium-enriched soy milk

1½ cups steamed butternut squash cut into small cubes
⅓ cup raw cashews
2 shallots and/or chives, finely chopped
1½ cups your choice of chopped raw green vegetables
   (zucchini, broccoli, green beans, peas or green pepper)
Pinch of nutmeg
Fresh tarragon, dill or parsley
Paprika

Combine all piecrust ingredients and press into an ungreased pie dish.

Beat together the eggs and milk. Pour into the uncooked piecrust and sprinkle in the other ingredients. Flavor with fresh herbs such as tarragon, dill or parsley (if using dried herbs use sparingly as they are much stronger in flavor and can overpower the subtle flavors of this dish).

Sprinkle with a little paprika and bake in a moderate oven (350°F.) for 30 minutes.

Serves 6 (APPROXIMATELY 235 CALORIES PER SERVING)

QUICK CURRIED EGGS

4 hard-boiled eggs, sliced

SAUCE
2 teaspoons light margarine
1 tablespoon whole wheat flour
1 cup low-fat 2% calcium-enriched milk or soy milk
Mild curry spices to taste
Freshly ground black pepper
Chopped parsley to garnish

Arrange the sliced eggs in a shallow dish.

Melt the margarine over low heat and add the flour. Stir continuously for 1 minute until combined. Add the milk and continue stirring until the mixture boils and thickens. Add the curry spices and pour the mixture over the eggs. Sprinkle with the chopped parsley.

Serves 2 (225 CALORIES PER SERVING)

SLIMMERS' SPAGHETTI BOLOGNESE

2 onions, finely chopped
3 garlic cloves, minced
1 cup water
1 pound extra lean ground beef
½ green pepper, diced
15 ounces canned tomatoes
½ can condensed tomato soup (optional)
1 carrot, grated
1 celery stalk, chopped
Chopped mushrooms (optional)
2 bay leaves
Oregano or marjoram
Fresh parsley

Lightly cook the onions and garlic with water in a large saucepan (no oil). Add the beef and mix thoroughly with a fork to break up any lumps. Add the remaining ingredients and simmer with the lid on for about 1 hour. Remove the bay leaves and serve on the pasta of your choice.

Serves 8 (168 CALORIES PER SERVING; WITH 1 CUP PASTA 330 CALORIES PER SERVING)

POTATOES WITH SPINACH SAUCE

6 medium-sized scrubbed potatoes

SAUCE
2 teaspoons light margarine
1 tablespoon whole wheat flour
2 garlic cloves, minced
3 shallots, finely chopped
1 cup low-fat 2% calcium-enriched milk or soy milk
6 large spinach leaves, steamed and blended to a smooth puree
1 tablespoon pine nuts
Freshly ground black pepper

Poke holes in the potatoes with a metal skewer to enable faster cooking. Bake in a moderate oven or microwave until cooked through. Slice thinly and arrange in a shallow dish.

Melt the margarine and mix in the whole wheat flour, garlic and shallots. Stir over low heat for 1 minute. Add the milk and continue stirring until the mixture boils and thickens. Remove from the heat and add the pureed spinach, pine nuts and lots of black pepper. Pour over the potatoes and serve immediately.

Serves 6 (APPROXIMATELY 175 CALORIES PER SERVING)

LOW-CALORIE CANNELLONI

SAUCE
6 tomatoes, roughly chopped
2 shallots, finely chopped
1 small onion, finely chopped

½ green pepper, chopped
1 tablespoon chopped fresh basil
1 tablespoon chopped parsley
1 or 2 bay leaves

FILLING

6 to 8 spinach leaves, lightly steamed and roughly chopped
2 to 3 garlic cloves
1 onion, chopped
3 shallots and/or chives, chopped
½ cup chopped mushrooms
1 cup part-skim ricotta cheese
⅓ cup crumbled feta cheese
½ pound cannelloni shells (uncooked); buy shells that do not need to be boiled first

ALTERNATIVE CANNELLONI FILLING

6 to 8 spinach leaves, lightly steamed and chopped
2 carrots, grated
3 shallots and/or chives, finely chopped
2 teaspoons chopped fresh dill or ¾ teaspoon dried
2 avocados, coarsely chopped
1 cup mung bean sprouts

Place all the sauce ingredients in the microwave for 5 to 7 minutes or stir over moderate heat with no oil until cooked. (For your convenience, you may wish to purchase a fresh tomato sauce with similar ingredients and no added salt, preservatives or artificial additives and colors from your local supermarket.)

Combine all the filling ingredients in the blender and carefully fill the cannelloni shells.

Line the base of a shallow rectangular dish with a third of the sauce. Carefully place a layer of filled cannelloni shells onto this, covering the entire base. Top with the remaining sauce and bake in a moderate oven (350°F.) for approximately 40 minutes.

Serve with a large garden salad.

Serves 7 (APPROXIMATELY 200 CALORIES PER SERVING; APPROXIMATELY 245 CALORIES PER SERVING USING ALTERNATIVE FILLING)

AVOCADO PASTA

3 avocados
6 garlic cloves
½ cup fresh basil leaves
½ cup parsley
⅓ cup pine nuts
Freshly ground black pepper
Juice of ½ lemon

Blend all the ingredients together. Serve on the hot cooked pasta of your choice.

Serves 6 (APPROXIMATELY 465 CALORIES PER SERVING, INCLUDING 1 CUP PASTA)

EGGPLANT AND NAPOLITANA SAUCE FOR PASTA

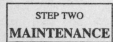

STEP TWO
MAINTENANCE

This is a delicious vegetable topping for pasta.

NAPOLITANA SAUCE
**2 cans peeled tomatoes or 8 to 10 tomatoes, chopped
½ green pepper, chopped
2 onions, chopped
Handful of chopped fresh basil
2 to 3 large eggplants
½ cup seasoned whole wheat flour
⅓ cup olive oil
¼ cup whole wheat bread crumbs
3 tablespoons sesame seeds**

Combine all the sauce ingredients in a saucepan and bring to a boil. Reduce the heat and simmer for 30 minutes, stirring occasionally to prevent burning.

Wash and slice the eggplants, sprinkle with salt and leave for 30 minutes. Place in a large colander and rinse off the salt under cold water. Pat dry and coat with the seasoned flour.

Heat a little oil in a nonstick pan and lightly fry the eggplant, being careful to drain well on absorbent paper.

Place a layer of eggplant in an ungreased casserole dish and top with a layer of basil sauce. Repeat this process, using alternate layers of eggplant and sauce until all the ingredients are used. Finish with a layer of sauce and sprinkle with whole wheat bread crumbs and sesame seeds. Bake in a moderate oven (350°F.) for 20 to 30 minutes.

Serves 6 (290 CALORIES PER SERVING EXCLUDING PASTA)

| STEP TWO |
| MAINTENANCE |

BARBECUED MARINATED SHRIMP

12 shrimp or prawns

MARINADE
2 tablespoons low-sodium soy sauce
1-inch piece gingerroot, sliced
3 garlic cloves, minced
2 fresh chilies, sliced
2 shallots, finely chopped
⅓ cup beer

Shell the shrimp, removing the heads but leaving the tails intact. Devein and wash them under cold water.

Mix all the ingredients for the marinade together in a dish and place the shrimp into this, making sure each shrimp is coated with the mixture. Leave for at least 1 hour.

Strain off the liquid and cook the shrimp, chili, garlic, shallot and ginger on the barbecue until they change color and are cooked through, about 7 to 10 minutes.

Serve with rice and salad.

Serves 4 (APPROXIMATELY 70 CALORIES PER SERVING)

| STEP TWO |
| MAINTENANCE |

GRILLED BEEF CURRY

3 pounds lean beef (eye round)
1 tablespoon ground coriander
1 teaspoon ground cumin
¼ teaspoon ground cardamom
½ teaspoon cinnamon

½ teaspoon ground black pepper
1 medium onion
3 lime or lemon leaves
1 tablespoon fresh gingerroot
3 garlic cloves
1 tablespoon cornstarch
1 tablespoon lemon juice

Trim all visible fat from the meat and cut into cubes. Combine all the dry herbs. Blend the onion, lime leaves, ginger, garlic, cornstarch and lemon juice until smooth. Add the dry herbs and blend again, making sure the mixture is well combined.

Mix the meat and curry paste together in a bowl, taking care to rub the paste well into the meat. Marinate for at least 1 hour (can be left covered overnight in the refrigerator).

The meat may then be threaded onto skewers and grilled or barbecued until tender.

Serve with rice and salad.

Serves 8 (APPROXIMATELY 355 CALORIES PER SERVING)

| STEP TWO MAINTENANCE | CHINESE STIR-FRIED VEGETABLES |

The addition of some sliced tofu to this dish will add more protein and calcium to this meal. Half a cup of tofu contains 130 mg of calcium.

½ green pepper
½ red pepper
2 medium carrots

2 medium zucchini
1 medium onion
4 shallots
1 bunch of broccoli
1 tablespoon light olive oil
1 teaspoon sesame oil
1 tablespoon fish sauce
20 raw cashew nuts
2 garlic cloves, chopped
1 tablespoon chopped fresh gingerroot
½ bunch fresh coriander, chopped
Fresh chili (optional)
Freshly ground black pepper
2 tablespoons ketchup manis (sweet soy sauce from an Asian shop)
4 tablespoons low-sodium soy sauce
1 small bunch of spinach

Prepare the vegetables and cut into large bite-sized pieces. Wipe the wok or large pan with a cloth dipped in olive oil so the stir-fry will not stick (a nonstick pan is better because you need no oil).

Place the sesame oil and fish sauce in the wok with ¼ cup water over moderate heat. Add the onion and cook until transparent. Then mix in the nuts, garlic, ginger, all the other vegetables, and pepper, except the spinach. Mix in the ketchup and soy sauce and more water if required, stirring constantly.

Break up the spinach leaves into small pieces and add just before the meal is ready to serve, as they require minimal cooking. All the vegetables should be slightly crunchy and the spinach should not lose its green color. Do not overcook.

Serve immediately with rice or noodles.

Serve 6 (APPROXIMATELY 120 CALORIES PER SERVING)

STEP TWO
MAINTENANCE CHICKPEA CURRY

2 onions
5 garlic cloves
2 teaspoons grated gingerroot
curry powder (or to taste)
1 cup coconut or soy milk
2 cups precooked chickpeas
2 tablespoons vinegar
2 tomatoes, chopped
1 cinnamon stick
1 tablespoon low-sodium soy sauce

Blend together the onion, garlic and ginger to a paste. Add the curry powder to the onion paste and continue to blend until they are also combined.

In a large saucepan, place a tablespoon of the milk and add the curry paste to this. Cook over moderate heat for 5 minutes, stirring constantly. Add the remaining milk, chickpeas, vinegar, tomatoes, cinnamon stick and soy sauce. Simmer for half an hour, stirring occasionally.

Serves 4 (APPROXIMATELY 250 CALORIES PER SERVING)

STEP TWO
MAINTENANCE CARIBBEAN CHICKEN

2 pounds skinless chicken thigh fillets, trimmed of fat
Paprika
2 garlic cloves, minced
3 small dried chilies, finely chopped

3 tablespoons honey
½ cup low-fat 2% calcium-enriched milk
2 tablespoons lime juice

Sprinkle the chicken fillets with paprika and grill until golden. Transfer the chicken to a casserole dish or saucepan. Combine all the other ingredients in a bowl and mix well. Pour over the chicken and cook over low to moderate heat for 25 minutes, turning the chicken and stirring occasionally. The sauce will reduce and thicken.

When serving, spoon the sauce over the chicken.

Serves 8 (APPROXIMATELY 250 CALORIES PER SERVING)

CHICKEN IN A PARCEL

2 chicken breasts
12 dried apricots, finely chopped
2 tablespoons plus ⅓ cup plain low-fat yogurt
2 tablespoons chopped walnuts or pecans
½ teaspoon thyme
Freshly ground black pepper
8 sheets filo pastry
2 tablespoons light margarine
1 tablespoon sesame seeds

Lightly pound the chicken breasts to an even thickness. Cut in half. Combine the apricots, 2 tablespoons yogurt, nuts and spices together and spread evenly onto each piece. Roll up quickly.

Brush one sheet of filo with a little of the extra yogurt and cover with a second sheet of pastry; brush again and fold in half to form a square. Place each chicken roll diagonally at the corner of a square of filo pastry, roll up into a pastry parcel, tucking the ends under as you go.

Place on a lightly greased baking tray and brush with a little melted margarine. Sprinkle with sesame seeds and bake in a moderate oven (350°F.) for 35 minutes, or until golden brown.

Serves 4 (350 CALORIES PER SERVING)

| STEP TWO |
| MAINTENANCE | TUNA BAKE

2 cups cooked brown rice
1 medium onion, chopped
2 celery stalks, chopped
Basic Foundation Sauce (page 184)
3 shallots, chopped
½ cup corn kernels
18 ounces tuna in spring water, drained
1 handful of parsley, chopped
3 medium potatoes, cooked and mashed
1 tablespoon bread crumbs and 1 tablespoon Parmesan cheese to sprinkle on top

Place the rice in the base of a large casserole dish. Lightly cook the onion and celery in a steamer or microwave to soften. Combine the sauce, onion, celery, shallots, corn, tuna and parsley and mix well. Pour over the rice and top with the mashed potato. Sprinkle with some bread crumbs and Parmesan cheese. Bake in a moderate oven (350°F.) for half an hour.

Serves 4 (APPROXIMATELY 525 CALORIES PER SERVING)

STEP TWO MAINTENANCE SALMON MORNAY

2 cups cooked pasta spirals
Mornay Sauce (page 195)
½ pound pink salmon, drained
1 small onion, finely chopped
2 shallots, finely chopped
Freshly ground black pepper
1 handful of chopped parsley
Juice of 1 lemon
½ green pepper, diced
¼ bread crumbs and ¼ cup Parmesan cheese for topping

Place the pasta in the base of a small casserole dish. Combine the sauce, salmon, onion, shallots, pepper, parsley, lemon juice and pepper and pour over the pasta. Sprinkle with the bread crumbs and Parmesan and bake in a moderate oven (350°F.) for approximately half an hour.

Serves 4 (APPROXIMATELY 350 CALORIES PER SERVING)

STEP TWO MAINTENANCE AUTHENTIC BOLOGNESE SAUCE

2 pounds extra lean ground beef
2 small onions
½ bunch of fresh basil
1 handful of Italian parsley
2 tablespoons olive oil (authentic but optional)
2 garlic cloves, minced

30 ounces canned tomatoes or equivalent fresh, chopped
3¾ cups tomato or V8 vegetable juice
4 tablespoons tomato paste
1 bay leaf
Freshly ground black pepper

In a large heavy saucepan, over low heat, brown the beef, squashing with a fork as you go to stop it from forming lumps. Blenderize the onions, basil and parsley and add to the meat, mixing well.

Next add the oil and garlic, followed by the tomatoes, V8 juice and tomato paste. Add the bay leaf and pepper and cook over low heat, stirring occasionally and shaking the pot. Cook for 35 to 45 minutes.

Serves 8 (APPROXIMATELY 340 CALORIES PER SERVING)

STEP TWO
MAINTENANCE

BLENDER CREPES

This is a slightly thick batter that, when cooked, is strong enough to hold fillings such as beef, chicken, rice or fish.

1 cup whole wheat flour
2 eggs
½ cup low-fat 2% calcium-enriched or soy milk
⅓ cup water
1 tablespoon light margarine, melted

Place the ingredients in a blender in the listed order. Blend for 30 seconds, stop and stir down the sides. Blend for 1 minute until the mixture is smooth. Cook in a nonstick frypan over moderate heat.

MAKES 12 CREPES (APPROXIMATELY 60 CALORIES PER SERVING)

STEP TWO	SAVORY FILLINGS
MAINTENANCE	FOR CREPES

Make Blender Crepes. Use your imagination and fill each crepe with your own combinations of sauces, herbs, vegetables, meat, seafood, poultry or cooked legumes.
Try these combinations:

- Mushroom Sauce (page 194), cooked brown rice, fresh tarragon, shallots and cubes of cooked chicken
- Mornay Sauce (page 195), cooked shrimp, avocado and fresh parsley
- Lightly steamed vegetables with Dahl (page 210) and raw cashews
- Quick Mexican Beans (page 209), Chili Sauce (page 192) and a little cottage cheese
- Egg Sauce (page 194), pureed spinach and fresh dill

Calories will differ according to amount of filling used. If low-fat fillings are used and you limit the serving size to 2 crepes per person, the caloric level will be suitable for Step Two—Maintenance Program.

SWEET TREATS

WHOLE WHEAT PANCAKES

1 egg
1 cup soy or low-fat 2% calcium-enriched milk
¾ cup whole wheat flour
½ teaspoon baking powder
1 teaspoon vanilla extract

Beat the egg with half the milk. Mix in half the flour, then the rest of the milk and flour alternately. Add the baking powder. Beat well, making sure there are no lumps. Add the vanilla extract and let the mixture stand for 15 minutes.

Prepare griddle or pan by melting a little butter or margarine in it and wiping clean with absorbent paper; otherwise use a nonstick pan.

Over moderate heat, pour ¾ cupfuls of mixture into the pan. The pancakes are ready to turn when bubbles appear over the top surface. Turn once and serve when cooked through.

MAKES 6 PANCAKES (APPROXIMATELY 90 CALORIES PER SERVING)

APPLE AND OAT BRAN MUFFINS

1 large apple, grated
1¼ cups rolled oats
¼ cup oat bran
2 tablespoons olive oil
¼ cup raisins
1 tablespoon chopped walnuts
Poppy seeds

Combine all the ingredients, except the poppy seeds, in a large bowl and mix well. Spoon into nonstick muffin pans and sprinkle with poppy seeds. Bake in a moderate oven (350°F.) for 25 minutes.

MAKES 8 MUFFINS (APPROXIMATELY 135 CALORIES EACH)

BANANA AND PECAN MUFFINS

2 medium bananas, mashed
2 tablespoons honey
2 tablespoons olive oil
½ teaspoon vanilla extract
1¼ cups whole wheat flour
1 teaspoon baking powder
1 tablespoon chopped pecan nuts
2 tablespoons sesame seeds

Mix the bananas, honey and oil in a large bowl. Fold in the remaining ingredients, except the sesame seeds, and mix lightly. Spoon into nonstick muffin pans and sprinkle with sesame seeds. Bake in a moderate oven (350°F.) for approximately 20 minutes.

MAKES 8 MUFFINS (APPROXIMATELY 170 CALORIES EACH)

BLUEBERRY MUFFINS

½ cup low-fat 2% calcium-enriched milk
¼ cup part-skim ricotta cheese
2 eggs
3 tablespoons light margarine
2 cups whole wheat flour
1½ teaspoons baking powder
½ cup oat bran
1 tablespoon sugar
2 cups blueberries

Blend together the milk, ricotta cheese and eggs. Melt the margarine and add to this mixture, then blend again.

Combine the dry ingredients in a large bowl. Make a well in the center, pour in the blended mixture and mix well.

Lastly, fold through the fresh blueberries. Spoon into nonstick muffin pans and bake in a moderate oven (350°F.) for 25 minutes, or until golden brown.

MAKES 18 MUFFINS (APPROXIMATELY 100 CALORIES PER MUFFIN)

BANANA CREAM

Bananas are rich in potassium, which is necessary for cellular and enzyme activity.

Peel and freeze ripe or overripe bananas.

When bananas are frozen solid, blenderize them well. The mixture becomes thick and creamy, resembling banana ice cream.

EACH MEDIUM-SIZED BANANA YIELDS 90 CALORIES.

ICED PEACH TREAT

This is delicious on a hot day or after a meal to clean the palate. It is low in calories and rich in vitamins C and A.

2 ripe or overripe peaches, frozen
1 egg white

When the peaches are frozen solid, blenderize with the egg white. Serve while the fruit still contains some ice crystals.

APPROXIMATELY 75 CALORIES PER PEACH

BERRY DELICIOUS

1 cup raspberries or berries of your choice
1 tablespoon honey
Juice of 1 orange
2 teaspoons gelatin
1 cup part-skim ricotta cheese
Extra fresh berries and mint to garnish

Heat the raspberries, honey and orange juice together until hot but not boiling. Dissolve the gelatin in a little hot water and mix through. Blend lightly with the ricotta cheese and place in individual serving dishes. Garnish with extra berries and mint.

Serves 4 (APPROXIMATELY 160 CALORIES PER SERVING)

STEP TWO
MAINTENANCE

MINTED PINEAPPLE SORBET

1 cup water
1 cup unsweetened pineapple juice
1 tablespoon chopped mint
¼ cup sugar
1 tablespoon lemon or lime juice
1 cup blended fresh pineapple
2 egg whites

Combine the water, juice, mint and sugar and boil for 3 minutes. Set aside to cool. When cool add the lemon juice and blended pineapple and mix well. Place in a freezer tray and partially freeze.

Whip the egg whites into a meringue and fold through the pineapple mixture. Refreeze.

Serves 8 (55 CALORIES PER SERVING)

STEP TWO
MAINTENANCE   BAKED RICE PUDDING

½ cup brown rice
2½ cups soy or low-fat 2% calcium-enriched milk
1 egg, beaten
2 teaspoons golden syrup
2 teaspoons grated lemon rind
Grated nutmeg

Soak the rice in the milk for half an hour in a small ovenproof dish. Mix in the egg, syrup and lemon rind. Sprinkle with the grated nutmeg and bake in a slow oven 250°F. to 300°F. for 2½ hours. Stir after 30 minutes.

Serves 4 (APPROXIMATELY 120 CALORIES PER SERVING)

STEP TWO   STRAWBERRY-MELON
MAINTENANCE   MOUSSE

Rich in vitamin C and fiber, this is a delicious option if you are craving sweets. If you serve it with 2 teaspoons of low-fat yogurt you only add about 30 calories and you increase your daily calcium intake by 100 mg.

1 tablespoon gelatin
½ cup hot water
1 cantaloupe, coarsely chopped
¼ cup loosely packed brown sugar (optional)
½ cup orange juice
1½ cups strawberries, finely chopped

Sprinkle the gelatin into the hot water and stir with a fork until dissolved. Add the water and gelatin to the cantaloupe, sugar and orange juice and blend until smooth and frothy.

Gently fold through the strawberries and pour into a large bowl or 4 individual bowls. Refrigerate until partially set, stir again, then return the mousse to the refrigerator until set.

Serves 4 (125 CALORIES PER SERVING OR 88 CALORIES WITHOUT SUGAR)

FRESH FRUIT SORBET

The addition of citrus in this recipe makes it tangy and refreshing to the palate. Count it as a daily fruit serving. Other fruits such as papaya, mango, melons and berries can be used in this recipe.

2 cups strawberries
1 tablespoon lime or lemon juice
2 egg whites
¼ cup sugar (or Equal for lower calories)

Blend the strawberries with the lime or lemon juice and pour into a freezer tray. Partially freeze until ice crystals start to form.

Whip the egg whites and sugar until the mixture forms peaks and fold through the fruit mixture. Refreeze until set.

4 servings: 80 CALORIES PER SERVING; 6 SERVINGS: 55 CALORIES PER SERVING

STEP TWO
MAINTENANCE

LEMON SELF-SAUCING PUDDING

1 tablespoon light margarine
⅓ cup sugar
2 eggs
2 level tablespoons whole wheat flour
Pinch of baking powder
2 teaspoons grated lemon rind
Juice from 1 large or 2 small lemons
1 cup low-fat 2% calcium-enriched or soy milk

Cream the margarine with the sugar. Separate the whites from the yolks of the eggs. Add the flour and baking powder to the margarine and sugar. Add the grated lemon rind, juice, yolks and milk; mix well. Beat the egg whites to a meringue and fold through the mixture.

Pour into a lightly greased small casserole dish. Stand this in a baking dish containing cold water.

Bake in a moderate oven (350°F.) for 40 minutes.

Serves 6 (APPROXIMATELY 150 CALORIES PER SERVING)

STEP TWO	
MAINTENANCE	APPLE CRUMBLE

4 tart cooking apples
½ teaspoon allspice
½ tablespoon sugar or honey
2 tablespoons water

CRUMBLE MIX
2 tablespoons rolled oats
1 tablespoon dried coconut
1 tablespoon whole wheat flour
2 teaspoons sugar
2 tablespoons low-fat yogurt

Peel, core and quarter the apples and stew them with the allspice, sugar and water until just cooked. Place them in an ovenproof dish.

In a small bowl, mix the dry crumble mix ingredients together and add just enough yogurt to bind the mixture together. The mixture should still be quite dry. Sprinkle evenly over the top of the apples and bake in a moderate oven (300°F.) without a lid until the crumble turns golden brown, about 20 to 30 minutes.

Serves 4 (APPROXIMATELY 145 CALORIES PER SERVING)

STEP TWO	CREAMY ALMOND
MAINTENANCE	PUDDING

¾ cup cold water
⅓ cup brown sugar

3 teaspoons gelatin
¾ cup boiling water
1¼ cups evaporated skimmed or soy milk
1 teaspoon almond extract
3 tablespoons slivered toasted almonds

Place the cold water in a dish and add the sugar. Sprinkle the gelatin on top and stir in as you add the boiling water. Keep stirring until the gelatin and sugar have dissolved. Add the milk and almond extract; mix thoroughly. Pour into a medium serving bowl or 4 individual dishes. Garnish with the almonds. Chill until firm.

Serves 4 (IF EVAPORATED MILK USED, 130 CALORIES PER SERVING, IF SOY MILK 100 CALORIES PER SERVING)

STEP TWO
MAINTENANCE POACHED PEARS

This recipe could also be made in the microwave and the pears filled with spoonfuls of a mixture of chopped prunes, ground ginger, chopped almonds or pecans and brown sugar.

½ cup water
½ cup pear juice (apple or orange may be used)
1-inch piece of cinnamon stick
1 crushed vanilla bean (optional)
3 pears, peeled, halved and cored

Place all the ingredients except the pears in a large pan and simmer gently for 10 minutes. Add the pears and cook until just soft; do not overcook. Remove the cinnamon stick and vanilla bean. Serve with Vanilla Yogurt Sauce (page 236) or Almond Custard Cream (recipe follows).

An alternative would be to use 1 teaspoon of rose water instead of the other spices.

Serves 6 (120 CALORIES PER SERVING, INCLUDING ¼ CUP ALMOND CUSTARD cream)

STEP TWO	ALMOND CUSTARD
MAINTENANCE	CREAM

1 egg
2 teaspoons honey
1 cup low-fat 2% calcium-enriched or soy milk
1 teaspoon cornstarch
1 teaspoon almond extract

Beat the egg and honey together until well combined. Save a little milk to combine with the cornstarch and heat the remainder of the milk over moderate heat until lukewarm. Add the honey and egg, stirring well. Blend the cornstarch with a little milk and add to the other ingredients. Stir constantly until the mixture boils and thickens. It should be the consistency of a thin custard. Remove from the heat and add the almond extract.

Serve hot or cold.

Serves 4 (50 TO 60 CALORIES PER SERVING)

> STEP TWO
> **MAINTENANCE**   FLAPJACKS

This recipe is rich in fiber, protein and calcium. Serve flap-jacks hot or cold with fresh fruit and yogurt toppings.

2 eggs
1 tablespoon brown sugar
4 tablespoons LSA (page 263)
½ cup water
1 cup whole wheat flour
1½ cups low-fat 2% calcium-enriched or soy milk
¾ teaspoon baking powder

Beat the eggs with the brown sugar and add the LSA and water; mix well. Fold in ½ cup of flour, then ½ cup of milk. Mix in the remaining flour and baking powder followed by the rest of the milk. Let stand for half an hour to thicken.

Cook tablespoonfuls in a nonstick pan, turning once when bubbles appear on top. The LSA contains linseed oil so you will find the more flapjacks you cook, the easier they are to turn.

MAKES 24 FLAPJACKS (APPROXIMATELY 50 CALORIES EACH)

TOPPINGS

STEP TWO
MAINTENANCE

VANILLA YOGURT SAUCE

1 egg, separated
1 tablespoon honey
1 cup low-fat plain acidophilus yogurt
½ teaspoon vanilla
Cinnamon or nutmeg, if desired

Combine the egg yolk, honey, yogurt, vanilla and spice, if using, and mix well. Beat the egg white until stiff and fold through the yogurt mixture. Serve fresh. (This mixture will not keep.)

Serves 4 (75 CALORIES PER SERVING)

FRESH PEACH SAUCE

This sauce is easily digested because it is rich in enzymes. It is an excellent source of vitamin C, vitamin A and calcium.

Pulp of 1 peach
2 teaspoons lime or lemon juice
1 teaspoon grated lemon rind
½ cup plain low-fat yogurt
½ teaspoon ground nutmeg or cinnamon

Blend the ingredients until smooth and serve immediately.

Serves 4 (30 CALORIES PER SERVING)

CHAPTER SIXTEEN

EATING TIPS THAT CAN SAVE YOUR LIFE

There is so much information available today that many women are confused when making decisions about their dietary needs.

This section will explain how to use your food as a healing tool. You can allow your food to be your medicine and by following my recommendations and adapting good eating habits, you are preventing illness and improving vitality, health and well-being.

I have done a great deal of research into this subject so I have included the latest breakthroughs and vital facts on nutrition that every woman, desirous of good health for herself and her family, must know.

CARBOHYDRATES

Carbohydrate foods have a very important role in your diet. They are nutritious and filling and are excellent foods for achieving successful weight loss.

The main carbohydrates present in foods are sugars, starches and cellulose. The sugars and starches are converted by enzymes in your digestive juices to **glucose**, your blood sugar. This is your primary energy source. The cellulose contributes very little energy but provides you with bulk and fiber for intestinal motility and improves elimination.

Some of your glucose is converted to **glycogen** and stored in your muscle tissue and your liver. When your blood sugar level is low, glucose can be released from glycogen back into the bloodstream to provide you with the energy you need.

> **The best sources of carbohydrates in your diet are whole grain breads and crackers, cereals and grains, legumes (dried peas, lentils and beans), nuts and seeds, pasta, starchy vegetables and fruits.**

They are more accurately called **complex carbohydrates**. This is because they have a complex molecular structure. **They are full of nutrients and are naturally low in fat.**

Complex carbohydrates are more satisfying because they usually require more chewing and therefore take longer to eat. They provide you with a slower release of energy over a longer period of time, which is great for people who are trying to lose weight.

By eating a diet high in complex carbohydrates you will not have the highs and lows associated with fluctuating blood sugar levels. This will also reduce your cravings for sweets.

> **Keeping a high level of complex carbohydrates in your diet and doing regular exercise will burn fat and achieve healthier weight loss.**

Diets low in complex carbohydrates cause us to lose weight quickly by the loss of fluid and lean muscle tissue. As soon as we break our diet the weight comes straight back. We need our lean muscle tissue to keep us firm, not flabby, and to support our skeleton. Good muscle tone means less lower back and neck problems.

The unhealthy sugars and starches are refined carbohydrates. These provide fast energy and usually no nutrients. Refined carbohydrates are white sugar, white flour and products made from these such as cakes, biscuits, sweets and white bread. When you eat these foods you get a sudden rise in blood sugar, followed by a rapid drop. This leaves you craving more sweets and can often cause fatigue, headache, nervousness and giddiness.

Research shows that a diet high in complex carbohydrates will protect you against many illnesses, including obesity, cancer, diabetes and heart disease.

By following our Body-Shaping Diet you will ensure that your diet is rich in healthy complex carbohydrates. You will achieve weight loss without losing energy and you will burn fat, not muscle tissue.

BREAD AND CRACKERS

While you are on the Body-Shaping Diet weight-loss program—Step One, I recommend that you have **three servings each day** from this food group. I have included a short list of desirable bread and crackers from which you may select freely. **If you do not have cereal for breakfast then you may increase your allowance to four servings.**

I recommend whole grain choices as this is the best way to increase your daily fiber intake. You will also boost your nutritional input because the outside husk of the grain contains those essential B group vitamins for a healthy nervous system. This part of the grain also contains zinc, which improves your memory and maintains healthy hair, skin and nails.

White flour products only provide you with starch, which gives you temporary energy and a feeling of fullness.

When selecting bread, try to avoid loaves made with white or bread flour. They tend to have very low levels of zinc and high levels of cadmium, which is a toxic trace mineral that can increase hypertension.

If you don't like the heaviness of many whole grain breads, then simply choose a lighter whole wheat or stone-ground loaf. Try not to limit yourself to wheat bread alone. There are some delicious loaves available made from rye, barley, corn and oats, to name a few.

> **If you would like to avoid yeast in bread then try a sourdough loaf or yeast-free pita bread.**

You and your family will all benefit from the added fiber and nutrition.

Select three or four servings per day from the list below.
1 SERVING = APPROXIMATELY 75 CALORIES
      1 slice whole grain bread
      ½ roll (1 ounce)—whole grain
      1 slice pumpernickel

½ whole grain muffin (2 ounces)
½ pita bread (1 ounce)
4 Finn Crisp
2 WASA multigrain crispbread
2 Kavli crispbread
2 Ryvita sesame crackers
3 whole wheat saltine crackers
4 rice crispbreads
2 rice cakes
8 rice crackers (unsalted)
1 large taco shell
½ small whole wheat scone
1 small whole grain pancake

On our Maintenance Program—Step Two, you will increase your bread intake by one more serving. This means you will have four servings each day from this group plus cereal.

CEREAL CHOICES

When you are selecting a breakfast cereal, take the time to read the product information on the packaging. You may be surprised to find that some popular brands have extremely high levels of fat, sodium and sugar.

I recommend that you choose from the following list:

¾ cup oatmeal	100 calories
½ cup barley	110 calories
½ cup brown rice	120 calories
2 Weetabix	94 calories
1 ounce Kellogg's Low Fat Granola	120 calories
1 ounce Quaker 100% Low Fat	110 calories
1 ounce Just Right	108 calories
1 ounce Balance	117 calories
1 ounce Low Fat Alpen	110 calories

1 ounce Komplete Natural Muesli	111 calories
1 ounce Familia No Added Sugar Muesli	100 calories
1 ounce Kölln Oat Bran Crunch	100 calories
1 ounce Kölln Crispy Oats	110 calories
1 ounce Fruit & Fibre Cereal	108 calories

MILK AND CALCIUM REQUIREMENTS

Generally speaking, women require 800 to 1000 mg of calcium daily. During pregnancy, lactation and menopause our calcium needs increase to 1100 to 1200 mg per day.

Every woman should check that her daily diet provides these amounts of calcium (see the table on the next page).

If your diet on any one day falls short of this, or if you are not sure, take a good-quality calcium tablet containing 600 mg of calcium every day.

One of the best sources of calcium is milk and you will see from the calcium table that a cup of milk daily will give you a good start to meeting your daily requirements. If you are following a dairy free diet and cannot drink cows' milk, you may choose goat or sheep milk products instead. These are good low-calorie alternatives and contain adequate amounts of calcium. (If you suffer from gas and cramping after consuming dairy foods, you may be lactose intolerant. Lactase, the enzyme needed to break down milk sugar [lactose], can be found in liquid and pill form in most supermarkets and when consumed along with dairy products may relieve unwanted symptoms. Lactose-reduced milks are also available in most supermarkets.)

You will see in the calcium table that some good soy milks, unfortunately, are not a good source of calcium. Therefore you will need to make sure your diet is supplemented with other foods rich in calcium or take a calcium tablet on retiring at night.

When choosing soy milk remember to carefully read the

GOOD CALCIUM FOODS

FOOD	AVERAGE SERVING	MILLIGRAMS OF CALCIUM
Whole milk	1 cup	300
Skim milk	1 cup	300
Lactaid nonfat milk, calcium fortified	1 cup	500
Easylac nonfat milk	1 cup	300
Nonfat buttermilk	1 cup	300
Goats' milk	1 cup	295
Creamy Original Vitasoy	1 cup	80
Rice milk	1 cup	2.5
Soy milk (unfortified)	1 cup	60
Soy milk (fortified)	1 cup	300
Powdered skim milk	1 tablespoon	130
Hi Calcium Borden	1 cup	1,000
VIVA (with extra calcium)	1 cup	500
Plain nonfat yogurt/ plain low-fat yogurt	6 to 8 ounces	240
Farmer or pot cheese	1 ounce	258
Feta cheese	1 ounce	129
Low-fat cottage cheese	1 ounce	35
Ricotta cheese	1 ounce	100
Egg (large)	2 ounces	35
Sardines	3.5 ounces	350
Salmon	3.5 ounces	190
Tuna (with bones)	3.5 ounces	290
Fish (fresh, cooked)	3.5 ounces	35
Almonds (unsalted)	1 ounce (25 nuts/ average)	70
Brazil nuts (unsalted)	1 ounce (7 to 8 nuts)	55

GOOD CALCIUM FOODS (cont'd.)

Food	Average serving	Milligrams of calcium
Walnuts (unsalted)	1 ounce (25 nuts/ average)	30
Pistachio nuts (unsalted)	1 ounce (23 nuts/ average)	40
Whole sesame seeds	1 ounce (2½ tablespoons)	290
Sunflower seeds	1 ounce (2½ tablespoons)	30
Rhubarb	half cup (cooked)	170
Orange	1	50
Cantaloupe	half	30
Fresh fruit	each piece (average)	10 to 30
Broccoli	1 cup	50
Spinach	1 cup	100
Vegetables	1 cup (average)	10 to 50
Chickpeas	½ cup	75
Baked beans	½ cup	60
Kidney beans	½ cup	60
Soybeans	½ cup	90
Bread (average all types)	1 slice	30
Cereal (average all types)	1 ounce	5 to 30
Tahini (sesame paste)	1 tablespoon	85
Hummus	1 tablespoon	15
Tofu	½ cup	130

contents of the milk on the packaging. Some soy products are high in sugar to make them more palatable. You can buy low-fat varieties of soy milk if you wish. I use soy in recipes as a substitute for cream or to give a creamy texture to sauces, soups or custards.

Rice Dream is a low-calorie beverage made from rice. Although it is a delicious and refreshing drink, it is low in calcium.

If you drink cows' milk then I recommend calcium-enriched milk.

SUGAR

While you are on Step One of the Body-Shaping Diet it is generally a good idea to avoid sugar that doesn't occur naturally in your food. The addition of sugar can quickly add unnecessary calories and it is easy to consume large amounts. One teaspoon of sugar contains about 20 calories and it has no essential nutrients. It doesn't satisfy your hunger and, in fact, once you start on sugar you may find that you will binge all day. This is particularly true for the gynecoid and thyroid body shapes.

Watch labels for high sugar levels in convenience foods such as soy milk, bottled sauces, spreads and canned foods. Remember that ingredients are listed in decreasing order of weight, so if sugar is listed first on the label then that food is chiefly made up of sugar. All ingredients ending in the suffix *ose* are sugars. Examples to watch for are sucrose, lactose, fructose, maltose and glucose. Other sugars are sorbitol and mannitol.

The difference between brown or black sugar and raw or white sugar is simply that it is less refined.

Molasses is a by-product of sugar refining and is the best choice of sweetener because it has slightly less calories than other sugars and the benefit of added nutrients, namely iron, calcium and potassium.

Honey is a very natural and pure product; however, it does contain the same amount of calories as sugar. The benefit of honey over sugar is that you tend to use less of it.

> When you have a craving for sweets try to satisfy it with small amounts of whole grain foods or fruit. This will be more satisfying and will stabilize your blood sugar level, eliminating the urge for sweets.

Sometimes cravings for sweet foods can be overwhelming. The supplements on pages 81 to 83 can reduce or prevent cravings for sugar and chocolates.

> It can be difficult to satisfy a craving for chocolate with a bowl of rice. Chances are that you are looking for comfort food rather than experiencing blood sugar fluctuations.
>
> Try having a cup of hot cocoa or carob (not hot chocolate), made with skim or soy milk and sweetened with a little honey, molasses or brown sugar. By doing this, you will satisfy the chocolate urge without all the added caffeine and fat.

ARTIFICIAL SWEETENERS

Artificial sweeteners are generally best avoided. They are chemically made and their long-term effects on health are still unknown.

Aspartame is a chemical found in some artificial sweeteners that can affect your nervous system by interfering with your ability to relax. **If you are high-strung and cannot get to sleep at night you should remove this from your diet.** Watch for hidden sodium in artificial sweeteners.

I do realize, though, that you may enjoy a soft drink occasionally or wish to make a sweet that is not going to add unwanted calories. In this case you should go ahead and not feel guilty about doing so.

THE SUGAR—FAT CONNECTION

Many overweight women do not like sugar alone; however, research has shown that when sugar is combined with cream, milk or fat, they love it.

Android-shaped women often tell me that if cakes and pastries are available to them, they will eat them, even though they don't necessarily enjoy them.

Sweet foods tend to be rich in fat and this is where the danger lurks. **Sugar makes fat more palatable and when it is added to high-fat foods it encourages the obese to consume more.**

Foods rich in sugar and fat will often replace nutritional foods in our diet, which can lead to vitamin and mineral deficiency.

If you are feeling like ice cream, then have sorbet made from fresh fruit, low-fat frozen yogurt, water-based Italian ices or tofu ice cream instead. They still contain sugar but it comes without the fat.

PROTEINS

Proteins are present in every cell of our bodies and are an important element in the growth, health and repair of all body tissues. This includes skin, hair, nails, internal organs, bones, cartilage, muscle tissue and blood.

They are also needed to manufacture hormones, enzymes for proper digestion and antibodies to fight infection.

During digestion, proteins within our food are broken down into simpler particles called amino acids. The amino acids are like building blocks that link together to form "human" protein, which can be used within our bodies.

Some amino acids are not manufactured by our bodies and must be provided in our foods. They are called the essential amino acids. They must all be present together, in the correct proportions, in order for our protein to be utilized.

Some foods meet our needs perfectly. We call them **complete protein** foods. They are mainly animal products such as meat, fish, poultry, eggs, milk and cheese. Soybeans are also a good source of protein and contain all the essential amino acids.

Foods that lack any one of the essential amino acids are called **incomplete proteins**. They are from plant sources and need to be combined in a meal to make sure you have the correct balance of amino acids.

Incomplete protein foods are grains, nuts, seeds, legumes (dried peas and beans), lentils, cereal, rice and pasta.

Combining protein is not difficult and it is very easy and safe to follow a vegetarian diet. It simply means that you would choose more than one food from this incomplete protein group with each meal.

So instead of having just lentils and vegetable, you would have lentils, brown rice and a vegetable. Some other examples are:

Cereal with soy or low-fat milk
Pasta with pesto sauce (contains pine nuts)
Tahini on whole wheat bread
Brown rice with lentils
Legumes with brown rice
Chickpeas with tahini (as in Hummus, page 171)

Some ready-made products that are complete protein foods are hummus, falafel, tofu, tempeh and other soy products.

Adding some soy, dairy products or eggs into your diet makes it easier to have the correct balance of amino acids. However, if you follow a strict vegetarian diet, you will need to take care with combinations.

If you are a meat eater, as a general rule, try to get two-thirds of your protein from plants and only one-third from animal sources.

PROTEIN REQUIREMENTS

Women require about 45 g of protein daily. This will alter slightly between the different body shapes. By following the eating plans in this book, you will be having the correct amount of protein for your body type.

Remember that your daily protein intake must be increased during adolescence, pregnancy and lactation

and be guided by your doctor or dietician during these times.

Here is a short list giving examples of protein levels in food:

3.5 ounces meat or poultry, cooked	= 30 g protein
3.5 ounces tuna	= 29 g protein
3.5 ounces salmon	= 20 g protein
1 egg	= 6 g protein
1 cup low-fat 2% calcium-enriched milk	= 12 g protein
1 cup soy milk	= 8 g protein
1 cup plain yogurt	= 8 g protein
½ cup baked beans	= 8 g protein
½ cup brown rice	= 3 g protein
½ cup soybeans	= 13 g protein
2 Weetabix	= 4 g protein
¾ cup cooked oats	= 3 g protein
1 slice whole grain bread	= 3 g protein

Try to obtain regular protein from plant and fish sources, not just land animals. This alone will ensure a low cholesterol level and a reduction in fats. Plant sources also provide us with additional carbohydrate and fiber.

HIGH-PROTEIN DIETS

When we eat more protein than we need, we store most of the excess as fat. The rest is converted to nitrogen and is flushed out of the body in the urine. As a result your urine can be loaded with ammonia and other toxic by-products. This can place unnecessary strain on the kidneys.

Research has shown that eating excessive amounts of protein has been linked to kidney disease, osteoporosis, heart disease and cancer.

Many athletes are led to believe that high-protein diets are best for them. This is not so. They need a diet rich in complex carbohydrates so their muscles are rich in glycogen. This will maintain a steady release of energy for stamina and endurance.

Don't forget, excess protein is not turned into muscle, it is turned into fat!

LEGUMES

Legumes include many varieties of lentils, peas and beans, such as red or brown lentils, chickpeas, black-eyed peas, pinto beans, navy beans, soybeans, light red kidney beans, red kidney beans, canellini beans and more. **They are all low in fat and rich in fiber, protein and carbohydrate, which make them an excellent substitute for meat in your diet.** All you have to remember is that some are incomplete proteins and as such need to be combined with other complementary protein foods.

For example, if you have a chickpea casserole, you would serve it with brown rice. A taco mixture made from kidney beans could be served with some plain yogurt. Lentil burgers can be rolled in sesame seeds and served on a whole wheat roll.

When you combine legumes with nuts, seeds, grains, cereal or dairy products you can be sure that your protein and nutritional needs are met.

Adding legumes to meat dishes will extend the meal, add fiber and improve its nutritional value.

Legumes are an economical food and they contain iron, thiamine (B1), riboflavin (B2) and niacin (B3). When they are sprouted, they are also an excellent source of vitamin C, and sprouted legumes are delicious and health promoting, so why not add them to your salads?

HOW TO COOK LEGUMES

Rinse the dried beans and place them in a large bowl with water (one cup beans to three cups water). Cover and soak overnight.

Another quicker method is to cover the beans with water and bring them to a boil. Boil for two minutes and remove from the heat. Cover and leave for one hour.

Soaking will retain the moisture that has been lost in the drying process. Unsoaked beans will be difficult to digest.

Brown lentils are much smaller than other legumes and only require minimal soaking.

Rinse the beans and place them in a saucepan of boiling water. You may wish to add some herbs, garlic or chopped onion to the water to add extra flavor. Do not add salt as this will make the beans tough. Reduce the heat and simmer for thirty minutes, or until the beans are soft and plump.

Old beans will take longer to cook. Drain the beans and proceed with the recipe.

If you are making a casserole, you can mix the presoaked beans directly into the dish, adding extra water or stock as required.

For convenience you may prefer to use canned beans. These have been prepared for you and require no soaking or precooking. Drain off their liquid and add these directly to your recipe.

FRUIT

People on weight-reducing diets must be careful to select foods that are high in nutritional value and not high in calories. Fruit is an excellent choice, providing us with essential vitamins, minerals and fiber.

Some fruits, such as pineapple and papaya, are rich in enzymes that assist our digestion and can help us absorb other nutrients. For example, if you wish to absorb more iron from your food simply serve the meal with fruit rich in vitamin C such as papaya, pineapple or citrus.

Always try to have fresh fruit that is in season. Juices are fine but often the pulp is left behind and this is needed to provide extra fiber. Fruit is more satisfying. You will be more likely to remain hungry if you just drink the juice.

The skin and white pith of citrus and some other fruits contain the bioflavonoids or vitamin P. They are essential for the proper absorption of vitamin C. They keep collagen (our intercellular cement) in a healthy condition and strengthen our blood capillaries. This prevents hemorrhages, ruptures of veins, bruising and slows down the aging process. Rutin is part of the bioflavonoids and is essential in the prevention and treatment of varicose conditions. Including this nutrient in your diet often elim-

inates tired aching legs. **Simply grate some of the rind when making citrus juices and add it to the drink.**

If you cannot get fresh fruit the next best choice would be frozen fruit followed by canned fruit in natural fruit juice. Dried fruits do not contain added sugar; however, they may have a preservative added to maintain the nutrients and some people may be sensitive to this. Dried fruits can also harbor molds, which need to be avoided if you have problems with allergies, vaginal thrush or candida. Remember that dried fruits have simply had the water removed so they are equal in calories to fresh fruit; it is easy to eat too many.

If you have problems with blood sugar levels, then eat your fruit with plain yogurt. You will find that this will sustain your blood sugar for a longer period and provide a sense of fullness.

A lack of fruit in the diet will lead to serious health problems. **Fruit is rich in nutrients and I recommend three to five servings of fruit daily.** Try not to exceed this amount.

Keep in mind that you must watch your intake of all foods, even the healthy ones. This is clear when we remind ourselves that cows can get fat by eating only grass.

FRUIT
SERVINGS

While on the Body-Shaping Diet—Step One, I recommend that you have only **three servings of fruit** each day.

When you move to the Maintenance Program—Step Two, you are allowed **five servings of fruit** each day.

FRESH FRUIT
EACH ONE OF THE FOLLOWING
= 50 TO 70 CALORIES
= 1 FRUIT SERVING

½ cup fresh fruit salad

½ medium to large banana

1 small apple or 4 ounces apple juice

2 kiwifruit

½ small papaya

½ cantaloupe/honeydew

½ large pear

¾ cup berries

20 small cherries

1 large fig

½ large grapefruit or 4 ounces unsweetened grapefruit juice

small bunch of grapes or 2.5 ounces grape juice

1 medium guava

6 small limes

3 small lemons

1 large or 2 small mandarin oranges

½ large or 1 small mango

1 medium orange or 4 ounces fresh juice

1 medium peach/nectarine

2 small slices fresh pineapple

2 small plums

2 starfruit (carambola)

1 cup strawberries

1 cup watermelon balls

1 small persimmon

1½ pomelos

1½ quinces

5 to 6 medium kumquats

3 fresh apricots

2 large pomegranates

½ cup canned fruit in natural juice

DRIED FRUIT
EACH ONE OF THE FOLLOWING
= 50 TO 70 CALORIES
= 1 FRUIT SERVING

6 pieces apple
4 pieces apricot
1½ tablespoons currants/
   raisins
3 pitted dates
1½ figs
4 prunes

3 strips mango
1½ tablespoons mixed fruit
   peel
1 ounce papaya spears
1 ounce peach
¾ ounce pear
¾ ounce pineapple

VEGETABLES

Fresh vegetables are a rich source of nutrients and fiber and contain no fat. Starchy vegetables like potato, sweet potato, carrots and beets are also a good source of carbohydrate to boost your energy levels and potassium, which regulates your fluid balance. Do not omit these vegetables in order to cut calories. **They are packed full of vitamins and minerals and are only fattening if they are cooked in or served with fat or oil.**

> The Body-Shaping Diet allows you to have unlimited green vegetables and salad. This is because they are low in calories and will actually speed your weight loss.

Watery green vegetables assist the digestion of other foods. Meat and dairy products are heavy foods that tend to move through your intestines slowly. The addition of green vegetables will add water, fiber and enzymes to improve your ability to break down these foods and speed their elimination.

Green vegetables are extremely rich in the B group vitamins. These are water soluble and vital in the breakdown of fats and the proper functioning of your nervous system.

> **Some B vitamins are destroyed at the boiling point and for this reason green vegetables must be eaten raw or steamed to retain these important nutrients. Take care if you microwave green vegetables that you do not exceed the boiling point.**

Yellow vegetables are an excellent source of vitamin A, a fat-soluble vitamin. Examples are carrots, sweet potato, pumpkin, parsnip, turnip and squash. Spinach, broccoli and beet greens also contain large amounts of vitamin A.

This vitamin maintains the health of your skin and the soft tissue that lines your digestive tract, kidneys and bladder. It reduces your susceptibility to infection and inflammation in these areas. Vitamin A also assists your eyesight and the health of your lungs, mouth, nose, throat and sinuses.

Cooking, mashing or pureeing yellow vegetables helps to release vitamin A from the cell membranes. It is more difficult to absorb and utilize this nutrient from raw food.

Vegetables that contain water-soluble vitamins are sensitive to cooking, whereas vegetables that contain fat-soluble vitamins need to be cooked to release the nutrients. This explains the importance of eating a **balance of raw and cooked food** in your diet.

For optimum nutrition choose fresh vegetables as your first choice, frozen vegetables next and canned vegetables last.

The best vegetables will be those that have been grown organically, picked ripe and eaten while still fresh.

FIBER

Some fiber is rough and visible like the husk around grain or the skin on fruit. We call this **insoluble fiber** because it will not dissolve. During digestion we cannot break it down with enzymes or gastric secretions. Instead it absorbs water and provides bulk to our feces. Our stools become softer and heavier, which allows them to move through our intestines faster. As a result we eliminate constipation and reduce the incidence of diverticulitis, appendicitis, bowel cancer, spastic colon, and hemorrhoids and other varicose conditions.

Other types of plant fiber may consist of gums, pectin and mucilages and this is called **soluble fiber**. It dissolves easily in water and is found in legumes, cereal, oat bran, fruits and vegetables. This soluble fiber protects us against gallstones, ulcerative colitis, Crohn's disease, high blood pressure, high blood cholesterol and diabetes.

Fiber is an important part of the Body-Shaping Diet because fiber fights fat and helps maintain hormone balance.

TOO MUCH FIBER?

Some people experience discomfort when they switch to a high-fiber diet. Try to persevere because symptoms should lessen after a few days.

Symptoms can include increased flatulence, bloating, irritation, nausea and diarrhea. This is often a result of the addition of wheat bran, which can be an irritant to the intestine. I suggest you do not use this product.

The Body-Shaping Diet is not for weight loss alone—more importantly the emphasis is on good health. We are encouraging foods that are soothing and protective to the digestive tract.

> **The reduction of meat products and the addition of foods rich in mucilage and vitamin A (rolled oats, yogurt, yellow fruits and vegetables) can heal an inflamed colon.**

If you have diverticulitis then you should avoid whole grain products, little nuts, muesli and seeds as they can become trapped or caught in the bowel pockets. You should, however, still have fiber in your diet.

MINIMIZE FATS AND OILS

There is no doubt that fats and oils in your diet will stop you from losing weight and will contribute to obesity. Where do you think the word *fattening* originated?

Dietary fat that is not burned as energy is immediately stored as fat in your body.

Fats and oils are extremely high in calories and will slow down your metabolic rate. They are difficult to digest and, if eaten in excess, may interfere with your ability to absorb nutrients from other foods.

Is it so surprising that you feel so sluggish and uncomfortable after eating foods with a high-fat content?

Many fats can be reduced in your diet simply by changing habits and cooking techniques.

A quick way to lessen the amount of fats in your diet is to stop buying processed foods. You know that packaged cookies, cakes, pastry and fried foods are full of fat.

Reducing fats in your diet will also reduce your risk of heart disease and cancer.

Start making healthy choices and feel the benefit.

TYPES OF FATS

SATURATED FATS

Saturated fats are solid at room temperature.

If you have a diet high in these fats you are more likely to have obesity and clogged arteries and you increase your risk of cancer of the breast, colon, ovaries and uterus.

Examples are fat in beef, pork, lamb, poultry, whole milk, cream, cheese, ice cream, chocolate, butter, meat drippings, suet, lard, coconut and palm oils.

UNSATURATED FATS

These are liquid or soft at room temperature.

Examples are fish oils, soft margarines, olive, linseed, canola, grapeseed, peanut, corn, safflower, sesame, soybean and sunflower oils.

These oils are a combination of monounsaturated and polyunsaturated oils.

The best choices of these oils are olive, canola or linseed. This is because these oils are predominantly monounsaturated oils.

Research shows that small quantities of these oils can be beneficial to the health of our arteries. They can be used as salad dressings or in small amounts for cooking. There is no need to supplement your diet with more than this.

High-fat diets containing polyunsaturated oils and saturated fats have been shown to increase cancer growth in laboratory animals. So too have low-fat diets containing polyunsaturated oils.

There is no evidence at this time of any links between monounsaturated oils and cancer growth.

None of these fats and oils are healthy if we subject them to heat processing or if we fry food in them!

MARGARINE OR BUTTER?

There is a great deal of debate and confusion regarding the use of butter or margarine.

Butter is a saturated fat and as such should be avoided if you are trying to achieve weight loss and/or reduce cholesterol levels.

The lymphatic, gynecoid and android body types must avoid butter completely and only use a light, reduced-salt margarine that is dairy free. In the early stages of weight loss they may need to avoid butter and margarine completely.

The thyroid body type will metabolize cholesterol foods better than the other body types and may include butter if they wish.

Margarine is a man-made product and many brands contain excessive chemicals to make them look and taste like butter. When analyzed, this doesn't sound terribly healthy for us at all. We recommend Promise, Fleischmann, Mazola or any canola oil–based margarine.

I suggest you try to avoid butter and margarine when following the weight-loss program—Step One. Your body will be provided with enough healthy oils from your daily allowance of nuts, seeds, grains and vegetable oils.

The addition of butter or margarine in your diet can quickly add unwanted calories.

1 level teaspoon butter	= 36 calories
1 level teaspoon margarine	= 36 calories
1 level teaspoon light margarine	= 18 calories

Try to eat sandwiches with tahini, avocado or hummus instead of margarine and butter.

LINSEED OIL—A WISE CHOICE

Linseeds, like evening primrose oil, provide your body with some healthy omega 6 essential fatty acids and fiber. The following mixture can be made at home or purchased from a health food outlet.

**LSA   =   LINSEEDS (3 PARTS)
SUNFLOWER SEEDS (2 PARTS)
ALMONDS (1 PART)**

   MIX AND GRIND TOGETHER INTO A FINE MEAL.

This is an excellent source of protein and contains calcium, phosphorus, potassium, iron, magnesium, copper, manganese, selenium, vitamin E, B group vitamins and vitamin A.

The linseed also has a laxative effect and this combination is an excellent addition to breakfast cereal, blended fruit shakes and can be added to many recipes to increase their nutritional value.

This mixture should always be purchased fresh (if already made at a health food store) and stored in your refrigerator.

1 tablespoon LSA   =   65 calories

CHOLESTEROL

Cholesterol is a pearly, fatlike substance that is produced in your liver. It cannot dissolve in water or blood and is transported in your body by lipoproteins. If your dietary cholesterol is high it may end up being deposited on the walls of your arteries. High-density lipoproteins are scavengers and help to clean up this cholesterol and carry it back to your liver to be reused.

You can't eat these lipoproteins because they are not found in foods. However, you may increase the level of high-density lipoproteins by exercising, eating wisely, maintaining a healthy weight and not smoking.

Your body can produce all the cholesterol you need for health purposes without the need for added dietary cholesterol.

By having low dietary cholesterol, your need for high-density lipoproteins is also low. Generally it is ideal to have a blood cholesterol level of less than 200 mg/100 ml. Between 200 and 239 mg/100 ml is considered borderline high and over 240 mg/100 ml is considered to be a risk factor for cardiovascular disease. So I encourage you to keep your cholesterol levels at less than the 200 level. All the Body-Shaping Diets are designed to keep your cholesterol in the healthy range.

Obesity also increases the risk of heart disease so a restriction in dietary fat is necessary on both counts.

While following the Body-Shaping Diet you will benefit from a regime that is low in all fats and oils.

Reducing dietary saturated fat is only one of the methods of reducing cholesterol levels. Foods rich in saturated fats are all land animal products, including full-fat dairy foods, shellfish, coconut milk and palm oil.

You must also **increase foods** that will help to lower cholesterol. They include **vitamin C rich foods, garlic, onion and foods containing soluble fiber** (page 259).

Read the labels on packaged food carefully for fat content.

SALT—
SODIUM CHLORIDE

Salt is a compound of two elements, sodium and chloride. Forty percent of salt is sodium and this is the mineral that we will discuss in this chapter.

Let's start by outlining that sodium deficiency is extremely rare, due to the fact that sodium is found in all foods except fruit.

Our nutritional requirement for sodium is only about 250 to 350 mg each day. If one level teaspoon of salt contains 2000 mg of sodium then it is easy to see why so many Americans eat too much salt.

It is not so surprising when you consider how much salt is added to processed and convenience foods or what a standard addition to the dinner table is the salt shaker.

Your taste buds become accustomed to the flavor of salt. In fact, eating large amounts of salt can damage your taste buds and you may not be experiencing the true flavors of your food.

There are several things you need to do in order to reduce your sodium level. Read food labels and avoid those products that contain salt or sodium in any form. Watch for hidden sodium in the form of flavor enhancers and preservatives like monosodium glutamate or MSG. Occasionally it is included in salt shakers at fast food outlets and adds a slightly different flavor to chips and chicken. Artificial sweeteners can also contain high levels of sodium.

Reducing your intake of processed and fast foods usually leads to a large reduction of dietary sodium levels.

Stop adding salt to your cooking and put away the salt shaker. At first you will miss the salty taste. In fact you may have strong cravings for several weeks but they will pass. If you can persevere, after a couple of months your taste buds will come to life and you will be able to taste the true flavors of food once again.

> People with high blood pressure or fluid retention are usually advised by their health practitioner to reduce their salt intake. This is because research has shown a strong connection between these disorders and high dietary sodium levels.

The Body-Shaping Diet allows you to add roasted nuts, seeds, herbs, tasty sauces and low-calorie dressings to your food. If you are a salt user, the addition of these flavorings will help you to overcome the need to add salt.

TEA AND COFFEE

The Body-Shaping Diet allows you up to four cups of tea or coffee daily.

If you can only drink tea or coffee with sugar it might be wiser to avoid it unless you can become used to drinking it without. Or you may prefer herbal tea, which can be taken more freely and is easier to drink without sweeteners.

For tea drinkers I recommend that you limit tannin-containing tea to two cups per day. Tannin is a strong astringent and it can reduce your body's ability to absorb iron, which can lead to anemia.

Two brands of tannin-free tea that come to mind are

Celestial Seasonings and Lipton Soothing Moments. They are readily available at the supermarket or health food store and even hardened tea drinkers will be delighted with their flavor. Red bush tea is also delicious and has a similar taste to tannin tea.

Coffee is a stimulant that contains high levels of caffeine. If you enjoy a cup of coffee and have no bad effects from it, then 2 to 4 cups a day will not be harmful to you.

> Sensitivity to caffeine can bring on palpitations, anxiety attacks and migraine headaches. It can raise blood pressure, interfere with healthy sleeping patterns and weaken the muscle tone of your bladder. If you have any of these problems you should avoid coffee and other foods that contain caffeine such as cola drinks, chocolate and tea.

Women with lumpy, sore breasts will benefit by removing caffeine from their diet.

The alternatives are dandelion or cereal beverages, which contain no caffeine and are excellent coffee alternatives. Otherwise drink decaffeinated coffee.

Do not include tea or coffee when you calculate your daily water consumption.

ALCOHOL

Alcohol is hideously fattening so it can be extremely difficult to achieve weight loss, maintain good health and include alcohol in your regime all at the same time. Alcohol is very high in calories compared to other sources of energy. It yields 7 calories per gram compared to protein or carbohy-drate foods, which yield 4 calories per gram.

For women, one or two alcoholic drinks a day should not pose any serious health problems. However, you must reduce alcohol in order to lose body fat.

Remember that alcohol is a depressant that slows down the speed at which you digest food. It is also destructive to the nutrients and can reduce your calcium levels, paving the way for osteoporosis.

Even though it may be part of your social habits, I encourage you to say no. A couple of drinks may weaken your resolve and you are more likely to eat the wrong foods or, more seriously, substitute alcohol for food.

Once you reach Step Two—Maintenance, you may intro-duce one or two alcoholic drinks a day if you wish, although we do not recommend this. One or two drinks on the weekend is safe.

For now, eliminate alcohol and know that you are not adding empty calories. Instead, replace it with water, mineral water or seltzer with a twist of lime or lemon, or a fresh fruit juice.

ABDOMINAL SWELLING AND DIGESTIVE DISCOMFORT

Many women complain of fullness or bloating after eating. There is often an increase in gas or flatulence and occasion-ally pain or burning. This may be caused by physical prob-lems such as hiatus hernia, enzyme insufficiency or inflammatory disorders such as colitis, diverticulitis or ulcer-ation. Other causes may be candida, stress, food intolerance and sometimes poor food combinations.

Listed below are some self-help ideas for some of these problems.

HIATUS HERNIA. Eat smaller meals. Do not fill your stomach with large quantities of food or liquids as this causes the stomach to balloon out and leads to discomfort and pain. Avoid beer and carbonated drinks. Do not drink with meals.

INFLAMMATORY DISORDERS. Do not allow yourself to have long periods without any food. Save your fruit servings for in-between meals.

Select foods that are rich in vitamin A, such as yellow fruits and vegetables, to heal and soothe the tissues. Eat foods that will soothe and protect the digestive tract such as rolled oats, yogurt, papaya, pumpkin, sweet potato and rice.

Do not drink tea, coffee or alcoholic beverages. Chew slippery elm tablets or take slippery elm powder, mixed to a paste with a little hot water, fifteen minutes before meals and once before bed.

Try one or two small glasses of cabbage juice daily.

GAS OR FLATULENCE. Do not rush meals and maintain good posture while eating. Try eliminating all fermented foods such as vinegars, soy sauce, etc. Remove all sugar and foods containing added sugar from your diet. Reduce your intake of yeast by eating yeast-free bread and eliminating alcohol.

Try eating your fruit before your meal rather than after and do not eat fruit with bread, such as banana or apple sandwiches. Some people find that combinations of tomato and bread or meat and bread can also lead to discomfort.

You may find that taking a supplement of digestive enzymes may help. They simply provide you with extra enzymes to assist the digestive processes.

Herbal teas that would help are chamomile, peppermint, ginger, aniseed, caraway, cinnamon, cloves, lemon balm and dill.

PART FOUR

MORE BODY-SHAPING STRATEGIES

CHAPTER SEVENTEEN

CELLULITE

Cellulite is the word used to describe the lumpy uneven type of fat that accumulates on the buttocks and limbs of many women. It is rather unsightly because it gives the tissues underlying the skin (subcutaneous tissues) an orange peel or cottage cheese look.

Cellulite has been studied by doctors for many years and it has been categorized by several medical names such as lipodystrophy, mesenchymal disease or liposclerosis.

If we compare cellulite fat to normal fat we find that in the former there are abnormal physical and chemical changes.

In women with cellulite, pinching of the skin produces a "mattress appearance," with bulging and pitting of the fatty layer. On deep palpation of this layer one may be able to feel tender nodules of fat trapped inside hardened connective tissue.

There are several causes of cellulite:

hereditary factors   **lymphatic factors**
intestinal factors   **hormonal factors**
circulatory factors   **lifestyle factors**

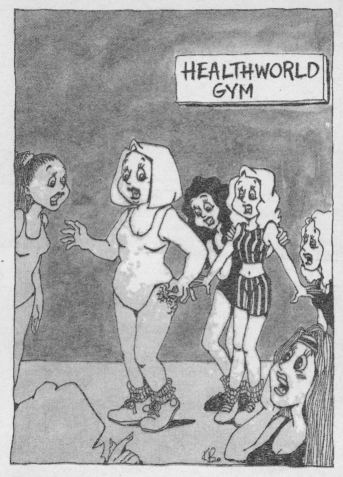

HEALTHWORLD GYM

The Body-Shaping Diet and exercise program takes all these factors into account and will gradually and efficiently eliminate cellulite.

Cellulite is most common in the gynecoid-shaped woman

Diagram 9

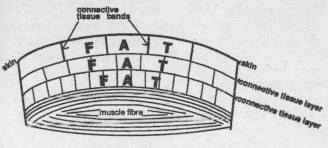

Anatomy of Fat Tissue
(note 3 layers of fat)

where it accumulates on the thighs and buttocks. In the lymphatic-shaped woman it accumulates on the legs, upper arms, buttocks and abdomen and is worsened by poor drainage of fluid through the swollen lymphatic vessels. If any of the four body shapes become overweight, cellulite may develop as the metabolism of the fatty tissues becomes increasingly underactive.

Diagram 9 shows us what normal fat tissue looks like under the microscope. If cellulite develops in fat tissue, it looks abnormal under the microscope and the fat cell chambers become swollen and pinched by the connective tissue bands seen in our diagram. This results in a restriction of the blood circulation through the tiny capillaries supplying the fat cells, which in turn reduces oxygen supply to the fat cells thus reducing their metabolism. This is why cellulite is so hard to lose. The connective tissue layers and bands become tougher and less elastic, trapping fluids and waste products between them and pinching the tiny ends of nerve fibers, which may cause areas affected by cellulite to ache. Eventually, in well-developed cellulite we see stagnation and hardening of all structures in the fat layers, so that the tissue takes on a lifeless quality—a bit like hard lumpy cheese.

To lose this cellulite the areas of fat affected must be revitalized and transformed, bringing back active metabolic processes within each fat cell. To achieve complete success we must have a plan of attack containing several strategies.

First, the Body-Shaping Diet should be followed for your particular body shape.

There are also some general strategies that must be applied for all body shapes afflicted with cellulite—that is, if they want to lose all their cellulite.

GENERAL STRATEGIES

Avoid saturated fats from fried foods, processed foods, full-fat dairy products, fatty meats such as pork, organ meats, lamb, commercially raised chickens, creamy or rich sauces and gravies, cakes and biscuits made with butter or processed fats.

Some women will find that their cellulite will not disappear completely while they continue to consume saturated fats. I remember one young woman with cellulite on her upper outer thighs that refused to budge while she continued with a diet containing three serving of low-fat dairy products daily. Only after eliminating all dairy products, red meats and chicken was she able to shed her cellulite.

If this is your case, then it is quite safe to completely eliminate all dairy products, red meats and chicken until your cellulite disappears. You are what you eat—if you are eating saturated fats and not metabolizing them, then they will be laid down as fat and perhaps cellulite in your body. Thus, for a limited time, until the cellulite disappears, you may need a diet free of all dairy products, red meat, and chicken.

While on such a diet, I advise a supplement of calcium

800 mg daily, organic iron 100 mg daily and vitamin B12 50 mcg daily. If you stick to a dairy- and meat-free diet for more than three months, please see your doctor to check your levels of vitamin B12 and iron.

For those wishing to lose cellulite quickly, the red meat-, chicken-free and dairy-free diet is superb. To make sure you do not become deficient in protein (in amino acids) I advise that you get first-class protein daily either from fish or by combining grains, nuts, seeds and legumes for at least one meal every day.

Avoid processed foods containing colorings, preservatives and flavorings, such as carbonated drinks, boxed and packaged cereals and meals, cakes and biscuits found in most supermarkets, foods made from white flour and sugar and foods high in salt.

Avoid alcohol—restrict your alcohol to one or two glasses on the weekend, or even better, avoid it completely.

Avoid snacks between meals—restrict these to raw celery, carrots or apples only and eat only three meals a day. Diabetics will need modification of this under supervision from their doctor.

Detoxify the body—the fat cells in cellulite are literally choked and suffocated by stagnant fluids and waste products trapped in hardened connective tissues. To transform these half-dead fat cells, we must first detoxify them or give them a "spring cleaning." This can be done by increasing your consumption of raw or living foods—such as sprouted seeds, raw fruits and vegetables. Some women prefer to do this by eating only raw fruits and vegetables for one or two days of every week—a type of raw food fasting, if you like.

Alternatively, you may elect to have a fruit-only breakfast, which is a great way to cleanse the liver and bowels for the start of the day.

I am often amazed by the number of women who rarely eat salads of raw vegetables except on hot summer days, as they see this as rabbit food and not the foundation of a

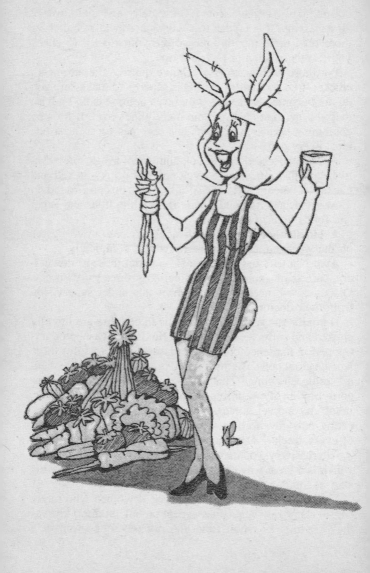

healthy diet. Our mothers and grandmothers often inculcated this misconception during our childhood.

My recommendation, not only for cellulite sufferers but for all women desirous of good health and a longer life span, is to eat one huge raw salad—full of fresh raw vegetables of all varieties—*every day*. Dressings can be made with lemon or lime juice or apple cider vinegar and a touch of cold pressed olive oil, sunflower, safflower or grapeseed oil. You may put avocado in your salads as it is free of cholesterol, two avocados per week being the maximum since it is high in fat.

To flavor the salads use fresh aromatic herbs and vegetables such as parsley, mint, coriander, basil, thyme, chives and/or finely chopped spring onions. A rather exotic taste to the salad can be obtained by using fresh ginger passed through a garlic press. For those who like more bite, use a dash of chili or soy sauce, garlic or black pepper.

The battle of cellulite will never be won unless you become a lover of raw foods every day. Make sure you chew slowly and thoroughly!

Another vital tool to detoxify and revitalize fatty tissues is to drink pure water—one and a half to two quarts daily is the target. This must be taken as water only or unsweetened herbal teas and not in the form of ordinary tea and coffee.

EXERCISES FOR CELLULITE

Exercise used as part of a program to reduce cellulite and help to keep it off needs to be **isotonic**. This means it needs to take you through a broad range of large movements such as in cycling, swimming, running, power walking or rowing. This kind of exercise shortens and lengthens your muscles rhythmically.

You need to become fit all over, which is why aerobic exercise, especially the low-impact type, is extremely beneficial for cellulite. The fitter you are the lower your resting heart rate is, which means you can deal better with stress without such a large buildup of chemical by-products in your system.

The best exercise is definitely a constant low-intensity, rhythmical type where you are using the large muscle groups at an intensity that increases your heart rate to 60 percent of your maximum heart rate—this is called your target heart rate and it is necessary to achieve this if you want to increase your metabolic rate and so increase the rate at which you burn up excess fat.

To find your **maximum heart rate,** subtract your age from 220.

To find your **target heart rate**, multiply the above figure (220 minus your age) by 0.6.

For example, if you are 40 years old your maximum heart rate = 220 minus 40 = 180 beats per minute. Your target heart rate = 180 × 0.6 = 108 beats per minute. By reaching your target heart rate via exercise you will increase your metabolic rate.

To reduce cellulite you should leave no longer than forty-eight hours between each session of exercise and you can work out for anything between thirty to sixty minutes a session, three to five times a week. Ideally, you could do five thirty-minute sessions as that would keep your metabolic rate up and running, therefore preventing the buildup of cellulite.

Massage and hydrotherapy are also excellent in helping to stimulate lymphatic drainage and reduce cellulite. Massage with an anticellulite preparation or essential oils can be very useful and should be done two to three times per week.

CHAPTER EIGHTEEN

EXERCISE

This is an essential part of your weight-loss and body-shaping program. Exercise will improve the health of your heart and lungs, regulate your desire for food and speed up your weight loss. Regular exercise greatly improves our moods because it stimulates the brain's production of endorphins, which are natural antidepressants. Your exercise routine should be done every day and if it is difficult to get out of the house you can do your exercise at home while listening to stimulating music. If you fall into the very overweight range, the best exercise to start with is gentle swimming or walking. As you lose weight more strenuous exercises such as aerobics or jogging can be started.

Be on the lookout for opportunities to exercise, such as getting off the bus a few stops earlier, taking the stairs instead of the elevator, leaving your car at home or taking a walk in the park at lunch. Some days you may feel like putting it off but try to force yourself to overcome laziness and lethargy because the results are many times worth the effort. The more you exercise the better you will look and feel. If you burn up 250 calories daily with exercise, this would result in a weekly weight loss of half a pound. If you

ACTIVITY	CALORIES BURNED PER MINUTE
Very light e.g. dusting slow walking, yoga	2
Moderate e.g. brisk walking energetic gardening scrubbing the floor	3.5–7
Heavy e.g. running, aerobics swimming laps, rowing weight training	>7.5

burn up 500 calories daily with exercise, this would result in a weekly weight loss of just over 1 pound.

BODY-SHAPING EXERCISE PROGRAM

The Body-Shaping Diet will allow you to lose weight from where you want to but we also encourage you to do a daily program of exercises designed to:

1. Warm you up.
2. Stretch and relax the muscles and joints.
3. Firm and tone the muscles so that your new shape will look firm and contoured.

By doing our simple and balanced exercise program you will be able to achieve your new body shape more quickly. Our exercises can be done in 20 to 30 minutes and should be done every day.

The exercises are designed for women who don't have a regular exercise program and you don't need to be fit to begin! If you have any medical problems it is wise to check with your doctor before you begin any exercise program. For those with any joint or back problems, consult a physical therapist who can modify these exercises specifically for you to avoid any injury or sprains. We also encourage you to do regular (2 to 3 times per week) recreational or aerobic exercise to promote overall cardiovascular and muscular fitness. Such exercises may include brisk walking, jogging, aerobics or sports such as rowing, tennis, basketball, scuba diving or golf. Tai chi or yoga can be very relaxing and improve muscular coordination, balance and posture. Aqua-aerobics or swimming are excellent exercises for all women but especially those with joint or back pain. Many a chronic backache has been cured with regular swimming alone.

One final word of warning—you should never force yourself to do or persist with any exercise that causes pain or discomfort.

WARM-UP

Take a brisk walk for at least 15 minutes daily, making sure that you relax the shoulders and swing your arms freely. Keep your body tall and straight and stretch the legs by taking large strides. Generally this will cause the pulse rate to rise to between 100 and 140 beats per minute. Count your pulse at the wrist for 10 seconds and multiply this number by 6 to give your pulse rate per minute. If you are a lymphatic type, walking is particularly beneficial in reducing swelling and puffiness of the legs and you should try to do 30 minutes of brisk walking daily.

STRETCHING—*for five minutes*

Stretching the muscles and joint ligaments in a gentle and gradual way will make you flexible and reduce sprains and injury. All exercises are to be repeated on each side.

1. Place one arm horizontally in front of your upper chest, flex it at the elbow and pull from the elbow to stretch the back of your arm and shoulder. Hold for 10 seconds.
2. Move your neck slowly to the right and then to the left— hold each side for 10 seconds.
3. Raise your arm behind your head and bend and stretch gently until the hand reaches the middle of your upper back—hold for 10 seconds.
4. Hold your foot against the corresponding buttock (bottom) to stretch the front of the thigh (quadriceps muscle)— hold for 10 seconds.
5. Lying with your back on the floor or on a rug, pull your leg toward your chest. It is important to keep your lower back flat and your head on the floor—hold this stretch for 10 seconds.
6. Lean your hands against the wall with your feet approximately 3 feet from the wall. Lean into the wall keeping your feet flat and feel your calf muscles stretch. Bend one knee forward toward the wall, keeping your back leg straight with its foot flat and toes pointed straight ahead. Press your heels to the floor and hold for 10 seconds.

EXERCISES TO STRENGTHEN, TONE AND FIRM THE MUSCLES

BOTTOM EXERCISES

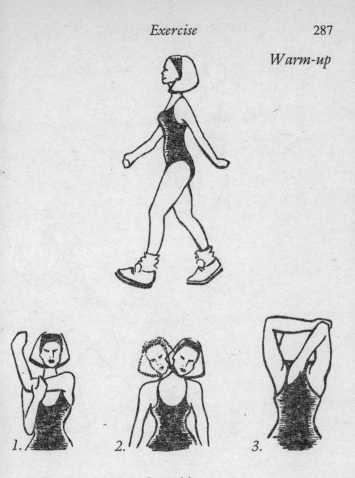

Stretching

1. Lie on your back with your knees bent and feet flat on the ground. Lift your bottom from the floor keeping your back straight. Do one set of 5 with feet apart and one set of 5 with feet together.

Stretching

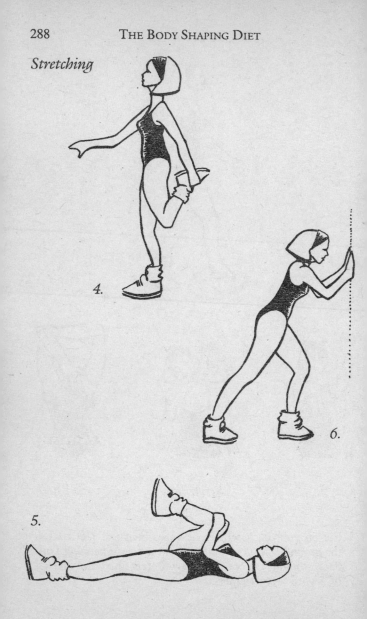

4.

6.

5.

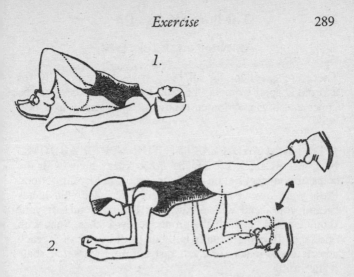

This exercise will firm and tone the muscles of the bottom and front thighs and is ideal for gynecoid-shaped woman. If you want to increase its effectiveness, do four sets of 5 (both feet apart and together) every day.

2. Get on your forearms and knees and keeping your back straight, stretch one leg backward, parallel to the floor, flexing your foot. Bring the knee forward under your stomach and then push the leg backward while holding in your stomach muscles. While the leg is back, bend it a little at the knee and lift it slightly (just 2 inches) skyward, keeping your foot flexed. Do 10 on each side.

This exercise firms the muscles of the bottom and back of the thighs (hamstrings) and is vital for women who want to reduce the size and floppiness of the back of their bottom. Gynecoid-shaped women should try to do 20 to 30 of these on each side.

ABDOMINAL EXERCISES

These are excellent for all body types but especially for android-shaped women who tend toward fat excess on the upper and lower abdomen (known disparagingly as a pot-belly).

1. TO FIRM AND FLATTEN THE UPPER ABDOMINAL MUSCLES. Lie on the floor, knees bent, with the soles of your feet flat on the floor and close to your bottom. Press your lower back into the floor and place your hands behind your head with elbows out behind you. Lift your shoulders and head off the ground a few inches. Start with one set of 10 and gradually build up to three sets of 10 each day. If tired, make sure you rest before each set. Exhale while lifting.

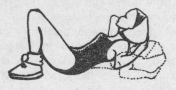

2. TO FIRM AND TONE THE LOWER ABDOMINAL MUSCLES. Lie on your back on a firm surface. Bend your knees and place your feet flat on the ground and your fingers next to your belly button. Raise one leg upward bringing your foot about 3 inches off the ground. Then lift up your other leg and hold both feet up for 5 to 10 seconds, then relax both feet back on the ground. Start with 10 of these and gradually build to three sets of 10 each day.

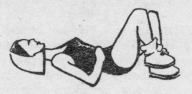

3. TO FIRM AND SHAPE THE WAIST. Sit on a stool and gradually tighten the stomach muscles until they feel tight and firm. Hold them tight for 5 to 10 seconds and then relax them while breathing out fully. Do this exercise 10 times and gradually increase it to three sets of 10 per day.

This is particularly beneficial for android and lymphatic-shaped women as it reduces a protuberant abdomen and encourages decongestion of the pelvic veins and lymphatic vessels.

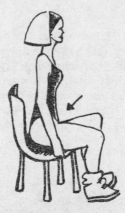

LEG EXERCISES

1. INNER THIGH. Lie on a firm surface and push your back into the ground. Bend your knees and place the soles of your feet together, still keeping your feet on the ground. Now squeeze your knees together and hold for 5 to 10 seconds. If this causes any discomfort on the knees, place a small folded towel between the knee joints to avoid pressure while squeezing them together. Start with one set of 5 working up to four sets of 5.

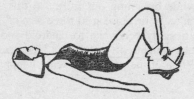

2. OUTER THIGH. Lie on your side on a firm surface with your upper leg straight and your lower leg bent at a 90-degree angle. Lift your upper leg straight up as high as possible, then slowly lower it. Keep your hips one above the other (i.e., don't lean forward or backward) and your toes pointing forward. Repeat lifting and lowering your upper leg 10 times, then roll over to the other side and repeat.

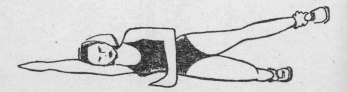

This exercise firms and tones the muscles of the buttocks and outer thighs and is great for gynecoid-shaped women wanting to reduce their bottoms and outer thighs.

ARMS AND CHEST

After losing weight many women find that the muscles of the back and the upper arm (triceps) remain loose and floppy. This can be avoided with these exercises.

1. Stand with one foot in front of the other, placing your body weight slightly forward. Bend your elbows, pressing them into the sides of your abdomen. Push each arm backward in a squeezing motion. Do one set of 10 and build up to three sets of 10 for each arm. You may find it comfortable to balance your body weight with a hand against a wall or on top of a dresser or bookshelf. This exercise can also be done using small handheld weights of 1 kg.

   This exercise is great for thyroid-shaped women wanting to build up their upper arms.

2. Sit on a stool, bring your arms up to shoulder height and bend the elbows. Slowly move the arms forward until the elbows and wrists touch in front of your chest and face, then move them back to the side, keeping them at shoulder height. Squeeze the arm muscles as you go. Start with 10 of these and gradually increase to three sets of 10.

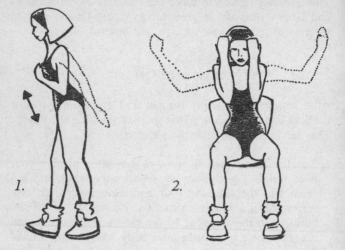

1.

2.

3. Begin on your hands and knees, with hands parallel to each other and a little more than shoulder width apart. The wider apart your hands are, the harder you will work your chest muscles. Lower your body, keeping it straight, until your chest only touches the floor, then push yourself straight up to the starting position. Repeat 5 times and gradually build up to 10 to 20 push-ups each day.

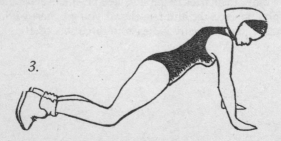

3.

CHAPTER NINETEEN

EATING DISORDERS

BULIMIA

Sarah was eighteen when she first discovered that making herself vomit was a way of controlling her weight. It was partly accidental—after a large meal she felt bloated and making herself vomit afterward seemed easy. It was the start, however, of a pattern of making herself vomit more and more often. She felt bad about doing it, hated being physically sick and began to avoid eating so she would not "have to" be sick. This meant that when she did eat she felt overly full very quickly and had an intense urge to vomit. She was vomiting three or four times every day by the time she decided she needed help to stop. She had difficulty coping with work and her part-time study because all her energy was used in thinking about eating and controlling her weight. She felt ashamed about her eating and vomiting and hated having to lie about it to keep it secret.

Sarah was suffering from bulimia, which today has become quite a common disorder in Western societies. Many of the features of bulimia overlap with those of anorexia but bulimic individuals tend to maintain their normal weight. When diagnosing bulimia doctors and psychologists have a technical definition that includes: a sense of lack of control, making yourself vomit, using laxatives or fluid tablets and strict dieting or exercising in order to prevent weight gain. People with bulimia also generally have an overconcern with body weight and shape similar to that seen in anorexia.

Apart from being unpleasant and distasteful, making yourself vomit is not an effective strategy for losing weight. Because it disrupts the body's natural way of obtaining nutrients from food, most people with bulimia develop other symptoms such as poor concentration, depression, moodiness, irritability and fatigue.

Repeated vomiting or purging can also be dangerous. The major medical risks come from changes in the body's natural salt balance, which commonly causes tiredness and muscle weakness but can also cause the heart to beat irregularly or even stop. Acid from the stomach also erodes tooth enamel and causes tooth decay.

Today there are many forms of treatment available. All involve learning something about the disorder and most involve coming to some understanding of the meaning of the illness for the individual.

Once the disorder is established it can be very difficult to stop by yourself and professional advice is generally the most reliable way of getting better.

Different therapists have different approaches and most will tailor the type of therapy to the needs and personality of the individual. It is important, firstly, to learn something about bulimia and about healthy patterns of eating and nutrition. A dietitian with experience in treating bulimia can be a great help with this. The most common psychological treatments involve a form of behavior therapy called cognitive behavior therapy. There are many elements to this but the focus of the treatment is on modifying the irrational thoughts that are associated with the binge eating and vomiting.

Many patients need to deal with painful feelings coming

from parts of their life unrelated directly to food, and other forms of psychotherapy may be most helpful for this. Bulimia is often exacerbated by life stress and learning other ways of dealing with this will generally be part of a treatment package. Your therapist will advise about the best treatment.

Some medications can be helpful for treating bulimia, particularly if depression is a major part of the problem.

Hospitalization in a specialized eating disorder unit is generally effective in breaking the bulimia cycle. Treatment in a hospital is essentially similar to that outlined above but is more intensive. It often involves group programs and allows eating behavior to be changed in a more structured way with twenty-four-hour support from experienced staff. Because in the long run the changes in behavior need to occur in the person's natural environment, hospitalization is generally reserved for people who are not able to solve the problem with outpatient treatment.

Without treatment, bulimia tends to continue over many years, often varying in severity in relation to stress. For some sufferers, the symptoms are quite incapacitating. A treatment program will usually take several months. Response to treatment is generally good, enabling people to get on with their lives without pervasive concerns about weight, shape and food.

This section on bulimia was written by Dr. Greg McKeough, a consultant psychiatrist who works with women suffering with eating disorders.

ANOREXIA NERVOSA— THE HUNGER WITHIN

Anorexia nervosa is the medical term for self-induced starvation. *Anorexia* means "loss of appetite" and the word *nervosa* indicates its relationship to an imbalance in the nervous system. In Westernized societies, anorexia nervosa is not an uncommon disorder. It affects one in every two hundred women under the age of twenty-five and typically has its onset in adolescence or the twenties. The anorexic woman becomes fully preoccupied with her body weight and shape and has a morbid fear of becoming fat. In many cases she would rather die than become fat! She pursues thinness relentlessly and fears food because she may not be able to control her weight if she eats one bit of food too much. Her rigid dieting is often accompanied by a rigorous schedule of arduous exercise that she forces herself to do in spite of her exhausted state. Eating may be followed by self-induced vomiting or ingestion of laxatives and purgative drugs. This can result in damaged teeth, swollen salivary glands and severe imbalances in body minerals.

I have called anorexia nervosa "the hunger within" because sufferers are not only starving physically but also deep inside their emotional being there is a hunger. They are hungry for love, acceptance, admiration, independence, maturity, indeed, for life. But they are in a paradox because although they want these things, they are too frightened to let themselves evolve and develop enough to grasp them. Fundamentally, the anorexic woman is terribly insecure, lacks confidence and has poor self-esteem, which makes it difficult for her to face the normal phases of life as she grows up. She may fear her sexuality and the prospects of sexual relationships, responsibility, childbirth or parenthood and tries to escape these things by starving herself into a childlike or preadolescent state. She wants to be a Peter Pan, never growing up and living in a fantasy world where she controls her life with a protective suit of armor in the form of childlike thinness. She regresses to a preadolescent physical state.

Her fear of womanhood and sexuality may be based on a poor relationship with her father, sexual abuse, incest or rejection from boyfriends or close friends.

Because adolescence brings the first prospects of independence and sexuality, it is not surprising that this is the most common time for anorexia nervosa to begin.

In general, the anorexic woman is resistant to help and does not go to a doctor of her own volition to seek treatment for her weight loss. In the majority of cases she is brought to a doctor by a family member or close friend who is concerned by her loss of appetite and weight. The anorexic woman usually makes light of her thinness and is evasive or untruthful in answering questions about her food intake. She will often state that she is still too fat and desires to lose more weight, even though to all others she appears painfully thin; this is due to her distorted body image.

PHYSICAL SIGNS

A woman suffering with severe anorexia nervosa will at some stage of her illness have the following physical signs of her disease:

1. A body weight of less than 80 percent of the average body weight for her age and height. In many cases she may weigh much less. Her body mass index will generally be less than 15.
2. Loss of regular menstrual periods due to her low levels of estrogen.
3. Soft downy hair growing on her limbs and face.
4. A slow heart rate, low blood pressure and cold hands and feet. This is due to a general slowing down of her metabolic rate, which occurs as a protective mechanism to slow down the rate at which her body consumes or lives off its own tissues.
5. Loss and wasting of muscular tissues.
6. Vitamin and mineral deficiencies.

TREATMENT

The aim of therapy is to restore body weight into the normal range. To do this it is necessary to supervise the food intake and in severe cases this is best done in a hospital that has a special program and inpatient eating disorder unit. Women with severe anorexia nervosa will usually spend eight to twelve weeks in a hospital.

Strategies that are helpful are individual counseling (psychotherapy), group therapy, nutritional counseling, body shape examinations, as well as analysis of eating behavior.

In severe cases forced feeding in hospital to save a life may be required. One can never be complacent or treat anorexia as a minor illness. It is a serious emotional and physical disorder that carries a significant risk of death.

Forced feeding will not provide a long-term solution and indeed patience and persistence are required because years of psychotherapy are often necessary to overcome anorexia nervosa.

During psychotherapy it is useful to explore childhood patterns of eating as there may have been a power struggle between the child and parents using food as the weapon. Other issues such as body image, self-esteem, expectations, assertiveness and sexuality need to be explored. Techniques of behavior modification, self-hypnosis, meditation and relaxation are useful to increase self-confidence and soften the high and often rigid standards that anorexic women impose upon themselves. Anorexic women may be obsessive perfectionists and they need to learn how to be kinder and gentler on themselves.

If the anorexia is associated with mental illness such as severe depression, psychosis or schizophrenia, antidepressant or tranquilizing drugs are required before other measures can be started.

The biggest hurdle to overcome is the resistance of the

anorexic woman to fully partake of the treatment program and that is why one in every ten anorexic women continues to be thin and unwell.

Women with anorexia nervosa can only use the Body-Shaping Diet under supervision from their doctor as they will need more calories than this to get their body mass index back into the normal range of 19 to 25.

NUTRITIONAL SUPPLEMENTS FOR WOMEN WITH EATING DISORDERS

Women with anorexia nervosa and bulimia have abnormalities in the function of their immune and hormonal systems. There are often imbalances in the chemical processes inside the body cells, with reduced energy production occurring.

Imbalances of this sort often cause fatigue, extreme mood changes, deep depressions, disturbed thoughts and cravings for refined sugars.

These symptoms can be greatly reduced by the regular daily ingestion of specific nutritional supplements.

Women with eating disorders need:

1. Niacin or niacinamide, 250 mg with each meal. This is also known as vitamin B3.
2. Essential fatty acids—with meals. Evening primrose oil, 2000–3000 mg daily. Fish oil 1000 mg daily.
3. Vitamin B complex, 1 daily with main meal.
4. Calcium, 1000 mg daily.
5. Iron amino acid chelate, 100 mg daily taken with vitamin C or citrus fruits.
6. Zinc chelate, 30–50 mg daily.
7. Vitamin B6 (pyridoxine), 50 mg daily with food.
8. Magnesium, 500 mg daily.
9. Vitamin C, 4000 mg daily.

The improvement that these nutritional supplements produce is truly remarkable and I cannot stress enough the importance of taking them regularly if you are a woman battling with an eating disorder.

For more information, contact:

American Anorexia and Bulimia Association, Inc.
133 Cedar Lane
Teaneck, NJ 07666
201-836-1800

National Association of Anorexia Nervosa and Associated
  Disorders
P.O. Box 7
Highland Park, IL 60035
708-831-3438

Anorexia Nervosa and Related Eating Disorders, Inc.
P.O. Box 5102
Eugene, OR 97405
503-344-1144

Bulimia, Anorexia Self Help
6125 Clayton Avenue, Suite 215
St. Louis, MO 63139
314-567-4080

National Anorexic Aid Society, Inc.
5796 Karl Road
Columbus, OH 43229
614-436-1112

Consumer Information Center
Dept. 551A
Pueblo, CO 81009
Brochure, "Eating Disorders," is free.

ADRENAL GLANDS Two small glands situated on top of the kidneys that secrete steroid hormones and the stress hormone adrenaline.

AMINO ACIDS The building blocks of the body's protein. Ten of the amino acids are essential dietary components as they cannot be synthesized by the body. Dietary protein can only be considered first class if it contains all the ten essential amino acids. First-class protein can be obtained from animal and dairy products and also by combining any three of the following at one meal: nuts, grains, seeds, legumes.

ANABOLIC STEROIDS Male hormones that stimulate the growth of bone and muscle.

ANDROGEN Male hormone.

ANOREXIA Loss of appetite.

ANOREXIA NERVOSA Loss of appetite and self-induced starvation due to an emotional illness.

ANTIMALE HORMONE A hormone that blocks the synthesis and effects of male hormones and is capable of reversing masculine body features.

ANTIOXIDANT Substances such as vitamins A, C and E, beta-carotene and selenium that protect the cellular structures from oxidative damage caused by free radicals.

BIOFLAVONOIDS Bioflavonoids are found in plants along with vitamin C and exert a beneficial effect upon the walls of the blood and lymphatic vessels. This is very helpful for women troubled with fluid retention and puffy limbs.

BODY MASS INDEX (BMI) The BMI is a scientific way of examining fatness and thinness and is worked out according to the formula BMI = weight/height squared. The normal BMI for women ranges from 19 to 25 kg/m^2 and many hormonal and menstrual problems can be overcome by keeping weight in the normal BMI range.

BODY TYPE There are four female body shapes or physiques, namely gynecoid, thyroid, android and lymphatic.

BULIMIA A disorder of eating characterized by lack of control, binge eating, making yourself vomit after eating, using laxatives, diuretics and strict dieting to prevent weight gain.

CAFFEINE A central nervous system stimulant found in tea, coffee and cola drinks.

CARDIOVASCULAR DISEASE Disease of the blood circulation system comprising the heart and blood vessels.

CHOLESTEROL A constituent of all animal fats and oils. It is found in the blood in two forms: 1. High-Density Lipoprotein (HDL), which protects against atherosclerosis, 2. Low-Density Lipoprotein (LDL), which promotes atherosclerosis.

COMPLEX CARBOHYDRATES Carbohydrates occurring in an unprocessed form and complexed with fiber, minerals and other nutrients. They are more slowly absorbed and utilized than processed or refined carbohydrates.

CORTISONE A steroid hormone made by the adrenal glands and also synthetically in laboratories. It improves well-being and has a powerful antiinflammatory effect.

DIURETIC A substance, whether synthetic or natural, that stimulates the kidneys to excrete salt (sodium chloride) and water, thereby relieving fluid retention.

ENDOCRINE GLANDS Glands that manufacture and secrete hormones.

ENDOCRINOLOGY The study and treatment of disorders of the glands and the hormones they secrete.

ENDOMETRIOSIS The presence of endometrium (which is normally confined inside the uterine cavity) outside of the uterus, scattered about inside the abdomen and pelvic cavities.

ENZYMES Proteins produced by living cells that function as catalysts in specific biochemical reactions.

ESSENTIAL FATTY ACIDS Fatty acids necessary for cellular metabolism that cannot be made by the body but must be supplied in the diet. Suitable sources are evening primrose oil, fish, fish oil, nuts, seeds and their oils.

ESTRADIOL A natural estrogen made by the ovaries. It is the most potent of all the natural estrogens.

ESTROGENS The female sex hormones secreted by the ovary being responsible for the female characteristics of breasts, feminine curves and menstruation.

EVENING PRIMROSE OIL The oil extracted from the beautiful evening primrose plant, which is renowned for its healing and tonifying properties. It is an excellent source of the omega 6 fatty acids, in particular the essential fatty acid known as gamma linolenic acid (GLA).

EXPECTORANT A substance that promotes the removal of mucus from the respiratory tract.

FEMALE SEX HORMONES The two sex hormones

produced by the female ovary—namely estrogen and progesterone.

FIBROIDS Noncancerous growths of the uterus consisting of muscle and fibrous tissue.

FRIENDLY PROGESTERONES Those type of progesterones that exert a favorable effect upon our blood vessels and skin and do not increase cholesterol, promote weight gain or masculine changes in the skin. Examples are cyproterone acetate, gestodene desogestrel, or natural progesterone.

GLANDS Organs or tissues, generally soft and fleshy in consistency, that manufacture and secrete or excrete hormones that exert their effect elsewhere in the body.

GYNECOLOGICAL ENDOCRINOLOGY Study of the hormones produced by women. It is a relatively new medical specialty that is expanding rapidly and brings the promise of exciting new developments and hope for many women.

HIRSUTISM A condition of excessive facial and body hair, excluding the scalp.

HORMONES Chemicals produced by various glands that are then transported around the body.

HORMONE REPLACEMENT THERAPY (HRT) The administration of hormonal preparations (natural or synthetic) to replace the loss of natural hormones produced by various glands.

HYPOTHALAMUS A major center situated at the base of the brain, regulating body temperature, thirst, appetite and other hormonal glands. It releases hormones that travel directly to the pituitary gland via a stalk.

IMMUNE SYSTEM The defense and surveillance system of the body that protects against infection by microorganisms and invasion by foreign proteins.

INFLAMMATION A condition characterized by swelling, redness, heat and pain in any tissue as a result of trauma, irritation, infection or imbalances in immune function.

INFUSION The process of steeping or soaking in a liquid to extract medicinal properties without boiling.

LYMPHATIC SYSTEM Drains fluid from the tissue spaces, transports fats and assists with immunity and our ability to overcome disease.

MALE HORMONE A hormone that promotes characteristics in the body such as facial and body hair, balding, acne, deepening of the voice and increased libido.

MENOPAUSE The final cessation of menstruation. The last period.

MENSTRUAL CYCLE The period of time from the first day of menstruation to the first day of the next menstruation.

METABOLIC RATE The rate at which the body converts food energy into kinetic energy.

METABOLISM Chemical processes utilizing the raw materials of nutrients, oxygen and vitamins along with enzymes to produce energy for bodily functions.

NATUROPATHIC MEDICINE The treatment of illness with naturally occurring substances such as organic foods, juices, nutritional supplements and herbs.

NONANDROGENIC Not causing masculine effects in the body.

OSTEOPOROSIS Loss of bone mass due to loss of bone minerals. Skeletal atrophy. Porous condition of bones.

OVARIES The female sex glands (gonads) located on each side of the uterus that produce eggs and the female sex hormones (estrogen and progesterone).

PITUITARY GLAND A mushroom-shaped gland connected by a vascular stalk to the base of the brain. The pituitary gland manufactures hormones, which in turn control other hormonal glands, such as the thyroid, adrenals, ovaries, testicles and breasts.

POLYCYSTIC OVARIAN SYNDROME A condition

of hormonal imbalance characterized by excessive male hormones and irregular menstruation. It is strongly inherited and may be triggered by stress or weight gain.

POLYCYSTIC OVARIES The type of ovaries present in women with polycystic ovarian syndrome. They have more than ten small follicles per ovary aligned around the edge of the ovary, whereas in a normal ovary they are distributed more evenly throughout the ovary. They can be seen by an ultrasound scan of the pelvis.

PREMENOPAUSAL The years, generally four to five, leading up to the menopause, characterized by a time of hormonal imbalance.

PROGESTOGENS Synthetic forms of the natural female hormone progesterone. They are commonly used in the OCP and HRT and regulate menstrual bleeding. Examples are norethinidrone, norgestrel and medroxy-progesterone acetate.

PROSTAGLANDINS Chemicals manufactured throughout the body that exert a hormonelike effect and influence muscular contraction, circulation and inflammation.

PSYCHOTHERAPY The treatment of mental and emotional imbalance through analysis of the thought processes, defense mechanisms and the subconscious mind.

SEX HORMONES The male and female hormones produced by the testicles, ovaries, adrenal glands and fat, e.g. estrogen, testosterone and progesterone.

STEROID DRUGS and HORMONES This group of hormones has a ringlike chemical structure. Examples of steroid hormones are cortisone and the male and female sex hormones.

SUBCUTANEOUS LAYER The fatty layer of tissue lying immediately underneath the skin.

SYNERGISTIC NUTRIENT A nutrient that helps or increases the effect of other body nutrients.

TANNIN Tannic acid—an astringent compound.

TESTOSTERONE The major male sex hormone.

THYROID GLAND The endocrine gland situated in front of the neck that produces the hormone thyroxine.

TONIC Producing and restoring normal tone and having the power to invigorate.

UTERUS The womb.

ULTRASOUND SCAN A method of visualizing the internal organs, fetus and blood vessels. Ultrasound does not incur any radiation exposure and utilizes very high frequency sound waves (more than 20000 hertz) that are above the audible limit.

Dr. Sandra Cabot, MBBS, DRCOG, is a medical doctor who has extensive clinical experience in helping women with weight problems, hormonal disorders and chronic health problems. A member of the Australian Council for Responsible Nutrition, she has helped many thousands of women through her several books, which are self-help guides explaining the tremendous power of nutritional medicine and natural hormone therapy. In this book, Sandra has combined her medical skills with the culinary skills of Australia's leading female naturopath, Deborah Cooper, ND Dip. Med. Herb., who is an expert at helping women with obesity, chronic health disorders and allergies to rediscover their lost form and health. Deborah's knowledge of nutritional medicine, food values, food combining and food preparation is as vast as it is inspiring. The Body-Shaping Diet menus have been Americanized by Johanna Burani, M.S., R.D., a registered dietician and nutrition educator and consultant based in New Jersey.

Dr. Sandra Cabot will be conducting seminars for women throughout the United States on The Body-Shaping Diet, and also on other women's health issues, including hormone replacement therapy and its alternatives, nutritional medicine, and hormonal imbalances, which can cause PMS, postpartum depression, acne, facial hair, headaches, decreased sex drive, and menopausal symptoms.

If you would like information about Dr. Cabot's upcoming seminars, or Dr. Sandra Cabot's Health Newsletter, which provides up-to-date information on both conventional and alternative healing techniques, or help in determining your body type simply send your name and address to:

Dr. Sandra Cabot
P.O. Box 1993
New York, NY 10113

Comments and questions regarding The Body-Shaping Diet can be sent to the same address.

I N D E X